FLORENCE NIGHTINGALE:
Saint, Reformer or Rebel?

FLORENCE NIGHTINGALE:
Saint, Reformer or Rebel?

RAYMOND G. HEBERT, Ph.D.

Associate Professor of History
Thomas More College
President, Kentucky Association of
    Teachers of History (KATH)

ROBERT E. KRIEGER PUBLISHING COMPANY
MALABAR, FLORIDA
1981

Original Edition 1981

Printed and Published by
ROBERT E. KRIEGER PUBLISHING COMPANY, INC.
KRIEGER DRIVE
MALABAR, FLORIDA 32950

Copyright © 1981 by
ROBERT E. KRIEGER PUBLISHING COMPANY, INC.

Printed in the United States of America

Library of Congress Cataloguing in Publication Data

Main entry under title:

Florence Nightingale—Saint, Reformer, or Rebel?

   Bibliography: p.
   1. Nightingale, Florence, 1820-1910—Addresses, essays,
lectures.   2. Nurses—England—Biography—Addresses,
essays, lectures.   I. Hebert, Raymond G., 1942-
[RT37.N5F56 1981]   610.73'092'4 [B]   80-28473
ISBN 0-89874-127-0

DEDICATION

for

MAUREEN, MICHELE and DANIELLE

the three strong, independent women in my life who supported my interest in, appreciation of and love for a fourth, Florence Nightingale.

Contents

FLORENCE NIGHTINGALE AND THE BIRTH OF
        PROFESSIONAL NURSING

FLORENCE NIGHTINGALE:
Saint, Reformer or Rebel?

Introduction

The name Florence Nightingale clearly symbolizes the nursing profession. Perhaps no name is better known by modern nurses. They have been told of the deplorable conditions in hospitals as recently as the mid-nineteenth century and concurrently how many of the revolutionary changes that followed the Crimean War (1854-1856) were due to the efforts of one woman—the miraculous, saintly "Lady with a Lamp," the "Angel of the Crimea." This portrait focuses narrowly on her Crimean War activities, portraying a composite Miss Nightingale as "the delicate maiden of high degree who threw aside the pleasures of a life of ease to succour the afflicted . . . gliding through the horrors of the hospital at Scutari [and] consecrating with the radiance of her goodness the dying soldier's couch." But, does this tell the entire story?

G. Lytton Strachey, for example, in 1918 disagreed with this uncritical portrait and reminded his readers that "the Miss Nightingale of fact was not as facile fancy painted her." Even Sir Edward Cook, however, in his classic 1913 two-volume study had striven to produce a human portrait rather than the "plaster saint" that had emerged from other sources. And, contemporary to the strong reaction against Strachey's iconoclastic approach, Mary Raymond Shipman Andrews, while proposing in 1929 that "a great commander was lost to England when Florence Nightingale was born a woman," did not neglect to point out that much of her success had been made possible because she was in fact so "quick, violent-tempered, positive, obstinate and stubborn." And even later, in 1951, Mrs. Cecil Woodham-Smith, in the tradition of Sir Edward Cook but with the Verney-Nightingale papers at her disposal, produced what most believe to be the first complete picture of Miss Nightingale—the woman of many faces with an abundance of faults as well as qualities.

Despite their efforts the earlier Crimean portrait, its narrow focus notwithstanding, still prevailed in the popular mind. As a result the full significance of her life was not appropriately recognized. As the articles in this collection will demonstrate, it is possible that her greatest contributions stem not from the Crimean War experience but from postwar

1

activities, her prodigious writings (200 books, articles, reports and over 12,000 letters) and especially her determination to create a profession. Little has been written in monograph form since the Woodham-Smith biography. However, an examination of the wealth of articles and papers that have appeared after 1951 permit a true picture of Florence Nightingale to emerge—not a saint certainly but no less effective because of what she accomplished as a reformer and "rebel with a cause." Evelyn R. Barritt, for example, in her 1973 article entitled "Florence Nightingale's Values and Modern Nursing Education" (*Nursing Forum*, XII, 1973), stresses how Miss Nightingale "made better health and better education her two objectives." In the process of building her case, Barritt introduces the reader to the highly-regarded but unpublished Stanford University dissertation by Mildred E. Newton. "Florence Nightingale's Philosophy of Life and Education" was completed in 1949. It emphasized how "deep religious convictions made service to God [Nightingale's] basic goal in life." She credits Miss Nightingale with five major accomplishments in addition to the precedent-setting Nightingale Training School at St. Thomas Hospital. These include: (1) improved and reformed laws affecting health, morals and the poor; (2) reformed hospitals and improved workhouses and infirmaries; (3) improved medicine—by instituting an army medical school and reorganizing the army medical department; (4) improved health for natives and British subjects in India and other colonies; and (5) established nursing as a profession with two missions—sick nursing and health nursing. In a similar view, Elmer Belt notes:*

> Her superior knowledge, her appreciation of social trends, the exactness and and truth of her statements, her dependability, availability and endless helpfulness endeared her to the leaders of her day. Her idealism, backed by positive demonstrable knowledge of human needs, brought about profound changes in their attitude toward general problems in human welfare. Through her influence a new humanitarianism was ushered in. To her originality we owe the vast public health programs which have resulted in better and healthier lives for all of us. The dreams of Florence Nightingale are today's realities.

As expressed by Evelyn Barritt, "Miss Nightingale's values for nursing education are viable today. Time provides an excellent test of values."

*Elmer Belt collected a valuable collection of Florence Nightingale materials that was then presented to the University of California Biomedical Library in honor of Dean Lulu Wolf Hassenplug for her successful creation of the school and its ten year direction. Kate T. Steinitz, Librarian of the Elmer Belt Library of Vinciana catalogued the collection and this work is available in the New York City Public Library.

But, if she can be remembered in some ways as timeless it is more important than ever to appreciate that this incredible woman was nonetheless Victorian.

Let us see how far, on the one hand, a sweet, shy, delicate flower of Victorian womanhood she was not and yet, on the other, the Queen who gave her name to the age honored her profusely and once said of her in what might be viewed as the ultimate compliment: "She has a wonderful, clear and comprehensive head. I wish we had her at the War Office."

Florence Nightingale was born on May 12, 1820, the younger daughter of William Edward and Frances Smith Nightingale. William was the wealthy son of a Sheffield banker and Frances was the daughter of the renowned early abolitionist William Smith. Stimulated by their wealth, they loved to travel and the only children, two daughters, were born during a long stay in Italy with both being named after their birthplaces. The elder, born in Naples during 1819, was named Frances Parthenope—Frances after her mother and Parthenope after the old Greek settlement on the site of Naples. The youngest was born at the Villa La Columbaia, Florence, Italy and accordingly named Florence.

The father Edward originally had Shore as a surname but, upon inheriting the Derbyshire estates of Lea Hurst and Woodend from his mother's uncle Peter Nightingale, he took the donor's name as well. Later, upon becoming High Sheriff in Hampshire, Edward purchased Embley Park there. The result was that much of Florence's early life was divided between Lea Hurst in the summers and Embley Park in the winters. Being a highly cultured country gentleman, this father of two bright daughters not only could accept but actually arranged for them to receive a liberal education. He personally taught them Greek, Latin, German, French, Italian, history and philosophy while a governess was brought in to teach music and drawing. The result, in Florence's case, was what some biographers describe as one of the best-educated women in Europe. The *London Times*, for example, in an October 30, 1854 story called "Who is Mrs. [Sic] Nightingale?" described her as a "young lady of singular endowments" with a "knowledge of the ancient languages, of the higher branches of mathematics, in general art, science and literature."

Nevertheless, it must not be forgotten that the life for a woman of status in the mid-Victorian world was rigidly circumscribed. "Delicacy" reigned and the women of her social class were restricted to society matters, appropriate entertainment and other such pursuits. Much was forbidden to women except what might be considered commonplace or trivial matters. Notably, however, these were the peaceful and prosperous years following the Napoleonic wars when new inventions abounded and great changes emerged in technology and the social realm alike. England's military and naval power enabled her to generate respect on land and sea. International trade flourished. The just and beloved reign of Queen Victoria, bolstered by the assistance of her beloved consort Albert, was symbolic of the place of Britain in international affairs. Through the first half of the century, "splendid isolation" was the predominant philosophy. Its success was reflected in the "Crystal Place" Exhibition of 1850.

But, if this world satisfied many, Florence Nightingale resented the self-abnegation that tied women of her social class to nothing more than "gentle sweetness." So frustrated was she in this futile, wasteful existence that she craved "for something worth doing"—escaping when possible into a world of her own. Many authors note that this desire to be somebody and do something useful was reinforced by a calling from God. One frequently-quoted note, written at the age of seventeen, read: "On February 7, 1837, God spoke to me and called me to His Service." Chafing, therefore, at the minimal opportunities open to a woman of her class, she developed a love of animals and the less fortunate. She began visiting many cottages to care for the sick. As reiterated by Newton and Barritt, it is clear that to Miss Nightingale, "serving God meant serving mankind." Soon afterwards, she began to visit a number of hospitals in London and the countryside. Her future was opening before her.

Secular nursing, however, was unfortunately one of the lowliest professions a Victorian woman could pursue. Generally placed on the level of a maid or menial drudge, nurses were a caste of questionable morals at best. The only respected nurses were those attached to a religious order. But there were too few of these and hospitals, in general, were only for soldiers, the poor or those affected by an epidemic disease. Charles Dickens was responsible for the generally-accepted stereotypes of nurses in the characters of Sairy Gamp and Betsy Prig—his "fair representation of the hired attendants on the poor in sickness." They were old, sloppy, careless, selfish and drunken. And, not only was the nursing considered to be beneath Florence's station in life, but was hardly even recognized as a work of mercy or philanthropy. Not surprisingly, any mention of interest in such an occupation was greeted negatively by her family. Fortunately, many contacts and friendships seemed to stimulate her during those difficult years: Sidney Herbert and his wife, neighbors at Wilton House in Hampshire; Chevalier Bunsen, the Prussian Ambassador to England and his wife; the American philanthropist Samuel Gridley Howe and his wife Julia Ward Howe and the Bracebridges, a group of traveling friends.

Yet, the 1840's were difficult years for Florence. In 1842, for example, she had asked some friends what could "an individual do towards lifting the load of suffering from the helpless and miserable?" By 1844 she seemingly had decided that her future lay in hospitals working with the sick. Consulting the much-respected Samuel Howe on this matter, he urged her to "go forward." From 1844 to 1851, meanwhile, she read voraciously, studied hospital reports, sanitary reports, materials describing the Kaiserswerth Institution in Germany, founded by Pastor Theodore Fliedner and his wife, Friederike. During all that time, however, the family quarreled openly and shamelessly over this determination of hers to become a nurse. Finally, in 1849-50, no doubt out of frustration, she left on a trip to Egypt with the Bracebridges. While stopping in Paris she observed the work of the Sisters of Charity. She recognized that their organization, discipline, attitude and sensitivity made them far better nurses than any in England. Conveniently, they gave her an introduction to their house in Alexandria where she inspected both their schools and hospital. On the way back, in the summer of 1850, she stopped off at the Institute of Protestant Deaconesses at Kaiserswerth on the Rhine near Dusseldorf. Pastor Fliedner's institute had grown since 1833 into a training school for nurses of the sick and for women teachers. Religiously-motivated, the institution emphasized simplicity and common sense. Though some biographers point out how later in life she spoke negatively about the quality of nursing there and described the hygiene as "horrible," this first visit nonetheless made a great impression on her. She returned to Kaiserswerth in 1851 and spent four months there (July to October) —completing a training course in sick nursing. Once back home, she wrote an anonymous account of Kaiserswerth entitled "The Institution of Kaiserswerth on the Rhine for the Practical Training of Deaconesses." She said later of that visit: "Never have I met with a higher love, a purer devotion, than there. There was no neglect. It was the more remarkable because many of the deaconesses had been only peasants: none were gentlewomen when I was there." The experience was clearly a turning point in her life.

More hospital visits followed during 1852-1853 (Edinburgh, Dublin, Paris). The objections of her mother and sister did not cease but to her credit she persevered. Though, at one point, while she was with the Sisters of Charity in Paris, the family called her back home to care for her dying grandmother. Quite tellingly, she returned without hesitation—family ties were still strong despite her purported rebellion. Soon after the grandmother's death she was asked to become Superintendent at the Institution for the Care of Sick Gentlewomen in Distressed Circumstances or the Harley Street Nursing Home. Though opposed to her interest in the position, once she began the duties her mother and sister accepted the inevitable—it had not been easy. While the position was but her first administrative post, many of her ideas were already revolutionary. She installed bells for the patients to ring if they needed help and lifts to hurry food to upper floors thus assuring that nurses could remain on the floors at all times. But her biggest challenge came from the Home's governing committee when she abolished the religious requirements for admission. They balked but the nursing care had improved so significantly during just one year that her ideas prevailed. She proved early that she would not be afraid to question authority and, in the process, provided a sample of what was possible through hard work and a willingness to experiment.

Following her one year commitment, all indications are that she was still dissatisfied. She had become acutely aware of deficiencies in hospitals everywhere and was not satisfied with her accomplishments in just one. So, after spending most of early 1854 at Middlesex Hospital, London, during a cholera epidemic she was more ready than ever to do what she could to alleviate problems on a broader scale. This explains, for example, why she expressed an interest in the superintendency at the more prestigious and newly-rebuilt King's College Hospital in London. Her highly-placed friend, Sidney Herbert, had already asked her to supply him with facts and figures to document what she called the sorry state of the pay and the accommodations for nurses. But, History had other plans for Florence Nightingale since, later in 1854, the Crimean War began. In 1853, a rekindled quarrel in Turkey, since dubbed the "Eastern Question," gave Russia the excuse to assert herself militarily. With England concerned over its crucial overland route to India, and France worried about its interests in the Holy Land both joined Turkey in opposing Russia. Because Russia had recently constructed a major sea base at Sebastopol in the Crimea this became the object of a joint British and French attack across the Black Sea through the Crimea. But, not only was the Crimea unknown to the allied armies when they arrived in September but the military strength of Russia had been underestimated as well. It was expected to be a quick punishing campaign. Instead, however, the incredible hardships of a Russian winter and multiple diseases, dragged it out into a full year of fruitless, degrading war.

The Crimean War, in fact, was almost totally dominated by blunders and mistakes—ranking undoubtedly as one of history's most useless wars. To begin with, no nation was really prepared for the war in general and in particular for supplying the armies in the Crimea. A disastrous cholera epidemic, with the accompanying lack of supplies, led to virtual chaos and disorganization. As British casualties mounted, for example, the Turkish government gave them the huge barracks at Scutari across the straits from Constantinople—this became the hospital for better or for worse, poorly equipped though it was.

As depicted by Sidney Godolphin Osborne in his *Scutari and its Hospitals*, the conditions were beyond imagination, with more deaths attributed to typhus, cholera and dysentery than to battle wounds. No man was more effective at informing the British public of this abominable situation than the *London Times'* Irish war correspondent, William Howard Russell. He was hated and certainly feared by generals and physicians alike and for good reason. He accurately reported many weaknesses and failures of the war effort. He exposed the inefficiency, corruption, idleness and incompetence that had crept into the British military since the days of fighting Napoleon in 1815. The English military establishment was solidly entrenched and self-protected. As a result, the fighting men were neglected, supplies were lost and there was no hope for the wounded, sick and starving.*

Noticing, however, that the Sisters of Charity and other religious made the conditions in the French hospitals far better than the British, Russell asked symbolically: "Why have we no Sisters of Charity?"

Russell's reports aroused horror and anger among the British public. Reacting immediately, Florence Nightingale, after gathering a group of nurses, wrote a letter offering their combined services to Sidney Herbert, the newly-appointed Secretary of War. Ironically, he had simultaneously reacted just as strongly, sending her a letter to ask if she would consider organizing just such a group willing to go to the front. He promised his complete support and assured her of sufficient supplies and personnel, medical and otherwise. Once she accepted he installed her as "Superintendent of the Female Nursing Establishment of the English General Hospitals in Turkey" and sent instructions to the commander-in-chief, Lord Raglan, the chief medical officer, Dr. John Hall and the purveyor-in-chief that they were to assist her in every way possible. Problems might have been anticipated, however, because the

---

*The extent of the incompetence, ill-preparedness and corruption is well-depicted in Mrs. Cecil Woodham—Smith's *The Reason Why* (London: McGraw-Hill, 1953).

military leaders blindly refused to admit that anything was wrong. The army medical department not only looked down on "women nurses" but felt threatened and resentful at this insertion of a well-placed friend of Secretary Herbert's in their midst. Both Herbert and Florence must have anticipated the worst because he authorized a commission of inquiry into the state of the hospitals and asked that Florence herself keep him well informed through regular reports.

On October 21, 1854 then, she, 38 nurses (10 Roman Catholic sisters, 8 Sisters of Mercy of the Church of England, 6 from St. John's Institute and 14 from various hospitals) and her friends the Brace-bridges left for the Crimea. They arrived on November 4, the eve of the disastrous unwelcome Battle of Inkerman. This part of Florence Nightingale's career is well known. Osborne spoke, for example, of the "complete absence of the commonest provision for the exigencies of the hour." The difficulties she faced cannot be exaggerated: the corrupt military and medical establishments, incredible conditions, inexperienced help or none at all. But, her "quiet resolution and dignity, her powers of organization and discipline rapidly worked a revolution" (*DNB*, p. 17). In the words of the already-quoted *London Times* article of October 30, 1854:

> While we write, this deliberate, sensitive and highly-endowed young lady is already at her post, rendering the holiest of women's charities to the sick, dying and convalescent. There is a heroism in dashing up the heights of Alma in defiance of death and all mortal opposition, and let all praise and honour be, as they are, bestowed upon it; but there is a quiet forecasting heroism and largeness of heart in this lady's resolute accumulation of the powers of consolation, and her devoted application of them, which rank as high and are at least as pure. A sage few will no doubt condemn, sneer at or pity an enthusiasm which to them seems eccentric or at best misplaced; but to the true heart of the country it will speak home, and be there felt, that there is not one of England's proudest and purest daughters who at this moment stands on as high a pinnacle as Florence Nightingale.

Florence Nightingale remained in the Crimea until August, 1856. The wounded had christened her "The Lady of the Lamp" and, as a sample of her work, a death rate at Scutari that had risen to 42% in February, 1855 was brought down to 2% in June of that same year. Henry Wadsworth Longfellow's poem, "Santa Filomena" accurately expresses the deep veneration that her courage and endurance, despite her own illness, had engendered. The other poem that symbolizes the

Crimean War is Alfred Lord Tennyson's "Charge of the Light Brigade." The failure and ineptness that it represents makes it easy to understand why she was welcomed back as such a heroine.

While a nation waited to shower her with admiration and laurels she characteristically returned quietly, her own health greatly impaired, to the family home at Lea Hurst. If anything, though, the haunting experiences of the Crimean War had convinced her more than ever that changes must be made. Some of her suggestions during the war had resulted in improvements, for example, in the training of medical personnel. Queen Victoria, meanwhile, showered her with multiple expressions of devotion. In January, 1856 she sent a personal letter of thanks with a beautiful, enamelled and jewelled brooch designed by the Prince Consort himself. It read "Blessed are the Merciful." The note ended: "It will be a very great satisfaction for me to make the acquaintance of one who had set so bright an example to our sex." And, in September of that same year, Florence visited Victoria at Balmoral, not missing the opportunity in the words of the Queen to "put before us all that affects our present military hospital system and the reforms that are needed: we are much pleased with her." Such powerful support along with the continued devotion and friendship of the ever-faithful and highly-placed Sidney Herbert led, for example, to the creation of a Royal Commission established "to examine the sanitary condition, administration and organization of barracks, military hospitals and the organization of the Army Medical Department." For this group she prepared a lengthy, confidential and privately printed report entitled "Notes on Matters Affecting the Administration of the Army" which included a Supplement on "The Introduction of Female Nursing into Military Hospitals in Peace and War." Significantly, this latter document had been requested personally by the Secretary of State for War, Lord Panmure, known not so affectionately by many as "the Bison." In this one case, as with many others, Miss Nightingale proved that "the Bison himself is bullyable."

Four subcommissions were generated by this Royal Commission's massive study and these smaller groups were authorized to carry out the reforms suggested by the commission. For many years, then, plagued by continuing ill-health,* she became nonetheless the authority on sanitary and hospital affairs, finding herself consulted routinely on all

---

*Upon her return from the Crimea it was diagnosed that her nervous system was ruined and heart affected, and that she would suffer routinely from recurrent spells and prostration. From the age of 36 on she was to remain confined almost exclusively to her bedchamber.

matters affecting Army health. Though in a confined environment, she filled her waking hours with blue books, reports and conversations with Sidney Herbert and the other members of her "Cabinet."* In time, she even made herself an expert on the sanitary needs of the Army in India.

Meanwhile, looking back to 1855, the only recognition for her great contribution that had been approved was the "Nightingale Fund," inaugurated for the sole purpose of opening a training school for nurses. By 1860 a £50,000 sum had already accumulated and some sources carry the final total to as high as £300,000. The result was the opening of the Nightingale School and Home for Nurses at St. Thomas Hospital, London. A handpicked choice, Sarah Wardroper, became the first Superintendent though Florence herself carefully monitored the progress and gave counsel, support and her personal touch on a regular basis. She cautioned, for example, that if women chose to enter a vocation, secular as well as religious, they must be as qualified as men. Much of her correspondence and many of her suggestions and addresses to graduating classes were printed for private circulation and therefore served as invaluable aids for the St. Thomas School and many others throughout the world.

She called upon her earlier successful experience in the Crimea where she had developed "eight fundamental principles regarding sound organization and administration" making them, in the words of Evelyn Barritt, the guidelines for her new school:

1. Certain goals or tasks require organized group effort, hence organization.
2. Each organization has a primary purpose.
3. Financial control provides administrative control.
4. Leadership of an area requires expertise in that area.
5. Hierarchical leadership roles with clear lines of authority and responsibility are needed.
6. Groups require clearly defined rules and regulations to function together as an organization.
7. Decision-making must be based upon the use of accurate data.
8. Efficient use of manpower is essential to an organization.

An example of her wide-ranging influence is the now-famous letter to Dr. Gill Wylie of Bellevue Hospital, New York City, in response to

---

*In addition to Sidney Herbert, several loyal, dedicated friends comprised what has been called her personal "Cabinet"—her brother-in-law, Harry Verney; Arthur Clough, the poet; Dr. Sutherland, a sanitary expert; and her Aunt Mai. Much of what she accomplished would not have been possible without their help.

his queries concerning a possible opening of the first such American Training School for Nurses. Miss Nightingale willingly and thoroughly answered all of his questions on such topics as the relationship that must exist between nurses and medical men, the importance of proper discipline and accordingly the need for a hierarchy of women culminating in the Superintendent, to whom "all reprimands" should be referred. Another indication of her thoroughness was the enclosure of an Appendix which specified "steps" that made up the training program at St. Thomas Hospital. The clear result of her work was that a profession had been created and the leap to the United States seemed guaranteed. Not surprisingly, in 1873, the first three American Nurse Training Schools were opened at Bellevue and also The Connecticut Training School in New Haven and the Boston Training School. At all three the Nightingale effort served as a model.

Incredibly, despite her interest in the school and its students and the time consumed by this mammoth undertaking, she still managed to accomplish much else as well. Most of this was done through her voluminous writings—letters, papers, reports, pamphlets and even books. Her most famous book, *Notes on Nursing*, originally published in 1860, is a special, timeless book that went through multiple editions even in her own lifetime and has just been re-issued once again in a modern version.* And, her equally-popular *Notes on Hospitals* (1859), which provides a myriad of details, arrangements and plans pertaining to civilian institutions, has also proven to be equally as lasting and invaluable. In short, for almost 45 years, this incredible woman, while "cooped up" in her sickroom, managed to spread many ideas and support her many causes through the power of the pen. It is therefore appropriate that Jean Nelson, in a 1976 article entitled "Florence the Legend" (*Nursing Mirror*, May 13, 1976), concludes that it is "daft" to think that Florence Nightingale can be understood and appreciated without reading her own words. To Nelson, therefore, "the power of the woman bursts from every page, and it is exciting reading for any nurse."

She was honored on numerous occasions even before her death— becoming a living legend. In 1907, for example, she was bestowed with the Order of Merit, "for outstanding intellectual prowess," by King Edward VII, the first time this honor had even been awarded to a woman. And, the following year, she received the Freedom of the City of London—this having been granted only once before to a woman, the

---

Notes on Nursing ed. by Muriel Skeet; foreword by Jean McFarlane, Edinburgh; New York, 1980.

Baroness Burdett-Coutts. Similar awards were received from France, Germany and Norway. Sadly, however, senility had set in during these last years so that the magnitude of this recognition may have been lost on her. Finally, during the last six months her sight, memory and eventually all sensation left her before death on August 13, 1910 at the age of ninety. She had asked for a simple burial so the family refused the government's offer of burial in Westminster Abbey. She was buried instead in the family's East Wellow, Hampshire plot. Also at her request, the inscription on the tombstone reads simply: "F.N. Born 1820. Died 1910."

It is this more multi-faceted woman, then, that emerges from the pages that follow. She was the powerful force who not only brought reform and improvements to nursing and nursing education but also to more far-reaching fields such as the army and medicine, public health, governmental legislation, statistics and especially the status of women. This is the impact expressed by Cook when he coined the phrase "Nightingale Power," meaning "Opportunity, Industry, Mental Grasp and Strength of Will." Or, by Woodham-Smith, when she concluded that "in the midst of the muddle and the filth, the agony and the defeats, she had brought about a revolution." Her greatest memorial, then, was clearly and appropriately her work—a realization best described by Stephen Paget for posterity in his *Dictionary of National Biography* article:

> Miss Nightingale raised the art of nursing in this country from a menial employment to an honoured vocation, she taught nurses to be ladies, and she brought ladies out of the bondage of idleness to be nurses. This, which was the aim of her life, was no fruit of her Crimean experience, although that experience enabled her to give effect to her purpose than were otherwise possible. Long before she went to the Crimea she felt deeply the "disgraceful antithesis" between Mrs. Gamp and a sister of mercy. The picture of her at Scutari is of a strong-willed, strong-nerved energetic woman, gentle and pitiful to the wounded, but always masterful among those with whom she worked. After the war she worked with no less zeal or resolution, and realized many of her early dreams. She was not only the reformer of nursing but a leader of women.

Not surprisingly, meanwhile, when an individual becomes a legend in one's own lifetime much of what makes up that legend is often the narrow perspective of an awe-struck author. The public's perception of a particular event or contribution often approaches the mythical.

Hence the emphasis over the years has been on Florence Nightingale as the "Angel of Mercy" or "Angel of the Crimea"; "Heroine of Mercy" or "Soldier's Heroine"; "Lady of the Lamp" or "Lady in Chief." Fortunately, however, the discriminating reader can also search harder and find the works that speak of her as a "Heroine of European Philanthropy," "Pioneer of Progress" or "Pioneer Among Women," "Lady with a Brain," "great religious thinker," "passionate statistician," "leader in religious thought and civic thought," "woman of renown" and ultimately "maker of history."

The articles selected for this anthology, then, are designed to show the depth and breadth of this remarkable woman. Looking at her within the context of her age and beyond she emerges as a full-fledged woman of the nineteenth century much influenced by that age and its problems in one sense, and as a woman for all time, timeless in her virtual singlehanded creation of a modern profession in another. Part I will initiate the reader to the plight of women in that early Victorian period. Charles Dickens' nurse stereotypes show the blatantly inferior pseudo-nurses Sairy Gamp and Betsy Prig with their open indifference to nursing standards. This is followed by Florence Nightingale's own bitter, impassioned 1852 essay on the plight of women in that era. Part II contrasts the 1910 portrait of Sir Edward Cook with that of the modern psycho-historian Donald Allen. This disparity will prepare the reader for the revelations of the articles that follow.

Part III, for example, provides a cross-section of descriptions about the well-documented and all-important Crimean experience. They include what many consider to have been the best of the Scutari eye-witness accounts. This is the description of Reverend Sidney Godolphin Osborne who attributed much of Miss Nightingale's success, curiously enough, to her "lively sense of the ridiculous." It is followed by a sample popular view that virtually sanctified her as one of the "heroines of modern progress," chapter 10 of what is clearly accepted as the standard biography by Mrs. Woodham-Smith, and is concluded with an excerpt from the opening chapter of a highly-praised new textbook, *The Advance of American Nursing* by Beatrice and Philip Kalisch. Part IV attempts to show how the post-Crimean exploits of Florence Nightingale were just as exciting and certainly more lasting than her accomplishments as the highly-publicized "Angel of the Crimea." It begins with Lytton Strachey's iconoclastic portrait that strongly rejects the popular saintly, delicate image and reveals instead a driven woman. In Strachey's words "she did not believe in gentle sweetness and womanly self-abnegation but strict discipline, rigid attention to detail, ceaseless labor, indomitable will with a cool and calm demeanor." The other articles, while less blunt than Strachey, nevertheless show what Florence Nightingale as author, reformer, and "rebel with a cause" believed in and accomplished.

And, finally, in the closing section, attention focuses on Florence Nightingale's role in the founding of a profession and on her timeless relationship to it. William Bishop tells of her "message for today"; two sociologists, Elvi Waik Whittaker and Virginia Olesen, see her unique contribution as nursing's legacy of status and prestige; Monica Baly describes convincingly how "no miasma of sentimentality nor subsequent reaction of anti-myth can destroy the solid facts of her achievements: they were Herculean"; and John D. Thompson, reflecting on her as a "passionate humanist," effectively traces the progress from "Nightingale to the New Nurse." Thompson, in this recent May 1980 article, states strongly that, in his estimation, the nursing profession is currently immersed in a serious dilemma. He notes the inability of nurses to agree internally on whether "nursing is a profession in and of itself, or whether nursing is a means to develop a better health care delivery system." And, in pursuing a solution, he suggests that the same issue "lies at the heart of the two faces Florence Nightingale has presented to posterity." Once again, in 1980, this foundress of a profession has many lessons for all who have followed in her footsteps. As A. G. Gardiner said in his *Prophets, Priests and Kings*: "She was not the Lady with the Lamp. She was the Lady with the Brain—one of those rare personalities who reshape the contours of life."

Begging your indulgence, as I conclude these introductory remarks, there are several select individuals and groups whose contributions must be acknowledged for without them this book would have remained but an idea. To the students of my History of Nursing classes back to the fall of 1978 who were so understanding about the hours spent attempting to find the real Florence Nightingale and who provided so much feedback and encouragement. To my colleagues in the History Department, Career Development Center and Learning Resource Center at Thomas More College who always understood what the study of Florence Nightingale and History of Nursing meant to me and cooperated accordingly again and again. To Mary Egbers whose typing skills, friendly smile and motherly demeanor carried me through my difficult times and Francis J. Bremer who as much as anybody else made me believe I could be an author. And, in a different but somehow deeper way, my parents, grandparents, wife Maureen and two daughters Michele and Danielle must be recognized because they never stopped believing in me. My grandmother Emma Landry, for example, who in her ninetieth year still demonstrates the "Nightingale Power" that Florence made so famous in her ninety years and my wife, Maureen, a modern nurse who reminds me constantly how the profession, if it is to not only survive but flourish and move forward, cannot settle for less than what this great pioneer and foundress believed in and fought for.

RAYMOND G. HEBERT
Thomas More College

June 1981

Nursing and the Plight of Women in Early Victorian England

Charles Dickens' *Martin Chuzzlewhit* (1843) has been thought to reflect the great nineteenth century novelist at his highest power (D.N.B.). This literary master's power of satirical portraiture and brilliance of style were all directed, he tells us, to one main object, "to exhibit in a variety of aspects the commonest of all the vices; to show how Selfishness propagates itself; and to what a grim giant it may grow, from small beginnings"(xvi). More specifically, in this excerpt from Chapter XV, none should doubt that his inimitable caricatures of the pseudo-nurses Sairy Gamp and Betsy Prig as "representations of the hired attendants on the poor in sickness"(xvii) demonstrate dramatically why nursing was considered an inferior and undesirable occupation.

CHARLES DICKENS (1812-1870)

Sairy Gamp and Betsy Prig Prevail

. . . She was a fat old woman, this Mrs. Gamp, with a husky voice and a moist eye, which she had a remarkable power of turning up, and only showing the white of it. Having very little neck, it cost her some trouble to look over herself, if one may say so, at those to whom she talked. She wore a very rusty black gown, rather the worse for snuff, and a shawl and bonnet to correspond. In these dilapidated articles of dress she had, on principle, arrayed herself, time out of mind, on such occasions as the present; for this at once expressed a decent amount of veneration for the deceased, and invited the next of kin to present her with a fresher suit of weeds: an appeal so frequently successful, that the very fetch and ghost of Mrs. Gamp, bonnet and all, might be seen hanging up, any hour in the day, in at least a dozen of the secondhand clothes shops about Holborn. The face of Mrs. Gamp—the nose in particular—was somewhat red and swollen, and it was difficult to enjoy her society without becoming conscious of a smell of spirits. Like most persons who have attained to great eminence in their profession, she took to hers very kindly; insomuch, that setting aside her natural predilections as a woman, she went to a lying-in or a laying-out with equal zest and relish. . . .

. . . 'Tell Mrs. Gamp to come upstairs,' said Mould. 'Now, Mrs. Gamp, what's *your* news?'

The lady in question was by this time in the door-way, curtseying to Mrs. Mould. At the same moment a peculiar fragrance was borne upon the breeze, as if a passing fairy had hiccoughed, and had previously been to a wine-vault.

Mrs. Gamp made no response to Mr. Mould, but curtsied to Mrs. Mould again, and held up her hands and eyes, as in a devout thanksgiving that she looked so well. She was neatly, but not gaudily attired, in the weeds she had worn when Mr. Pecksniff had the pleasure of making her acquaintance; and was perhaps the turning of a scale more snuffy.

'There are some happy creeturs,' Mrs. Gamp observed, 'as time runs back-ards with, and you are one, Mrs. Mould; not that he need do nothing except use you in his most owldacious way for years to come, I'm sure; for young you are and will be. I says to Mrs. Harris,' Mrs. Gamp continued, 'only t' other day; the last Monday evening fortnight as ever dawned upon this Piljian's Projiss of a mortal wale; I says to Mrs. Harris when she says to me, "Years and our trials, Mrs. Gamp, sets marks upon us all."—"Say not the words, Mrs. Harris, if you and me is to be continual friends, for sech is not the case. Mrs. Mould," I says, making so free, I will confess, as use the name,' (she curtsied here), '"is one of them that goes agen the obserwation straight; and never, Mrs. Harris, whilst I've a drop of breath to draw, will I set by, and not stand up, don't think it."—"I ast your pardon, ma'am," says Mrs. Harris, "and I humbly grant your grace; for if ever a woman lived as would see her feller-creeturs into fits to serve her friends, well do I know that woman's name is Sairey Gamp."'

At this point she was fain to stop for breath; and advantage may be taken of the circumstance, to state that a fearful mystery surrounded this lady of the name of Harris, whom no one in the circle of Mrs. Gamp's acquaintance had ever seen; neither did any human being know her place of residence, though Mrs. Gamp appeared on her own showing to be in constant communication with her. There were conflicting rumours on the subject; but the prevalent opinion was that she was a phantom of Mrs. Gamp's brain—as Messrs. Doe and Roe are fictions of the law—created for the express purpose of holding visionary dialogues with her on all manner of subjects, and invariably winding up with a compliment to the excellence of her nature.

'And likeways what a pleasure,' said Mrs. Gamp. turning a tearful smile towards the daughters, 'to see them two young ladies as I know'd afore a tooth in their pretty heads was cut, and have many a day seen— ah, the sweet, creeturs!—playing at berryins down in the shop, and follerin's the order-book to its long home in the iron safe! But that's all past and over, Mr. Mould'; as she thus got in a carefully regulated routine to that gentleman, she shook her head waggishly; 'That's all past and over now, sir, an't it?'

'Changes, Mrs. Gamp, changes!' returned the undertaker.

'More changes too, to come, afore we've done with changes, sir,' said Mrs. Gamp, nodding yet more waggishly than before. 'Young ladies with such faces thinks of something else besides berryins, don't they, sir?'

'I am sure I don't know, Mrs. Gamp,' said Mould, with a chuckle.— 'Not bad in Mrs. Gamp, my dear?'

'Oh yes, you do know, sir!' said Mrs. Gamp, 'and so does Mrs. Mould, your ansome pardner too, sir; and so do I, although the blessing of a daughter was deniged me; which if we had had one, Gamp would certainly have drunk its little shoes right off its feet, as with our precious boy he did, and arterwards send the child a errand to sell his wooden leg for any money it would fetch as matches in the rough, and bring it home in liquor: which was truly done beyond his years, for ev'ry in-dividgle penny that child lost at toss or buy for kidney ones; and come home arterwards quite bold, to break the news, and offering to drown himself if that would be a satisfaction to his parents.—Oh yes, you do know, sir,' said Mrs. Gamp, wiping her eye with her shawl, and resuming the thread of her discourse. 'There's something besides births and berryins in the newspapers, an't there, Mr. Mould?'

Mr. Mould winked at Mrs. Mould, whom he had by this time taken on his knee, and said: 'No doubt. A good deal more, Mrs. Gamp. Upon my life, Mrs. Gamp is very far from bad, my dear!'

'There's marryings, an't there, sir?' said Mrs. Gamp, while both the daughters blushed and tittered. 'Bless their precious hearts, and well they knows it! Well you know'd it too, and well did Mrs. Mould, when you was at their time of life! But my opinion is, you're all of one age now. For as to you and Mrs. Mould, sir, ever having grandchildren—'

'Oh! Fie, fie! Nonsense, Mrs. Gamp,' replied the undertaker. 'Devil-ish smart, though. Ca-pi-tal!' This was in a whisper. 'My dear—' aloud again—'Mrs. Gamp can drink a glass of rum. I dare say. Sit down, Mrs. Gamp, sit down.'

Mrs. Gamp took the chair that was nearest the door, and casting up her eyes towards the ceiling, feigned to be wholly insensible to the fact of a glass of rum being in preparation, until it was placed in her hand by one of the young ladies, when she exhibited the greatest surprise.

'A thing,' she said, 'as hardly ever, Mrs. Mould, occurs with me unless it is when I am indispoged, and find my half-a-pint of porte settling heavy on the chest. Mrs. Harris often and often says to me, "Sairey Gamp," she says, "you raly do amaze me!" "Mrs. Harris," I says to her, "why so? Give it a name, I beg." "Telling the truth then, ma'am," says Mrs. Harris, "and shaming him as shall be nameless betwixt you and me, never did I think till I know'd you, as any woman could sick-nurse and monthly likeways, on the little that you takes to drink." "Mrs. Harris," I says to her, "none on us knows what we can do till we tries; and wunst, when me and Gamp kept 'ouse, I thought so too. But now," I says, "my half-a-pint of porter fully satisfies; perwisin', Mrs. Harris, that it is brought reg'lar, and draw'd mild. Whether I sicks or monthlies, ma'am, I hope I does my duty, but I am but a poor woman, and I earns my living hard; therefore I *do* require it, which I makes confession, to be brought reg'lar and draw'd mild."'

The precise connection between these observations and the glass of rum, did not appear; for Mrs. Gamp proposing as a toast 'The best of lucks to all!' took off the dram in quite a scientific manner, without any further remarks.

'And what's your news, Mrs. Gamp?' asked Mould again, as that lady wiped her lips upon her shawl, and nibbled a corner off a soft biscuit, which she appeared to carry in her pocket as a provision against contingent drams. 'How's Mr. Chuffey?'

'Mr. Chuffey,' she replied, 'is jest as usual; he an't no better and he an't no worse. I take it very kind in the gentleman to have wrote up to you and said, "let Mrs. Gamp take care of him till I come home"; but ev'rythink he does is kind. There an't a many like him. If there was, we shouldn't want no churches.'

'What do you want to speak to me about, Mrs. Gamp?' said Mould, coming to the point.

'Jest this, sir,' Mrs. Gamp returned, 'with thanks to you for asking. There *is* a gent, sir, at the Bull in Holborn, as has been took ill there, and is bad abed. They have a day nurse as was recommended from Bartholomew's; and well I knows her, Mr. Mould, her name bein' Mrs. Prig, the best of creeturs. But she is otherways engaged at night, and they are in wants of night-watching; consequent she says to them, having reposed the greatest friendliness in me for twenty year, "The soberest person going, and the best of blessings in a sick room, is Mrs. Gamp. Send a boy to Kingsgate Street," she says, "and snap her up at any price, for Mrs. Gamp is worth her weight and more in goldian guineas." My landlord brings the message down to me, and says, "bein' in a light place where you are, and this job promising so well, why not unite the two?" "No, sir," I says, "not unbeknown to Mr. Mould, and therefore do not think it. But I will go to Mr. Mould," I says, "and ast him, if you like." ' Here she looked sideways at the undertaker, and came to a stop.

'Night-watching, eh?' said Mould, rubbing his chin.

'From eight o'clock till eight, sir. I will not deceive you,' Mrs. Gamp rejoined.

'And then go back, eh?' said Mould.

'Quite free then, sir, to attend to Mr. Chuffey. His ways bein' quiet, and his hours early, he'd be abed, sir, nearly all the time. I will not deny,' said Mrs. Gamp with meekness, 'that I am but a poor woman, and that the money is a object; but do not let that act upon you, Mr. Mould. Rich folks may ride on camels, but it an't so easy for 'em to see out of a needle's eye. This is my comfort, and I hope I knows it.'

'Well, Mrs. Gamp," observed Mould, 'I don't see any particular objection to your earning an honest penny under such circumstances. I should keep it quiet, I think, Mrs. Gamp. I wouldn't mention it to Mr. Chuzzlewit on his return, for instance, unless it were necessary, or he asked you point-blank.'

'The very words was on my lips, sir,' Mrs. Gamp rejoined. 'Suppoging that the gent should die, I hope I might take the liberty of saying as I know'd some one in the undertaking line, and yet give no offence to you, sir?'

'Certainly, Mrs. Gamp,' said Mould, with much condescension. 'You may casually remark, in such a case, that we do the thing pleasantly and in a great variety of styles, and are generally considered to make it as agreeable as possible to the feeling of the survivors. But don't obtrude it, don't obtrude it. Easy, easy! My dear, you may as well give Mrs. Gamp a card or two, if you please.'

Mrs. Gamp received them, and scenting no more rum in the wind (for the bottle was locked up again) rose to take her departure.

'Wishing ev'ry happiness to this happy family,' said Mrs. Gamp, 'with all my heart. Good arternoon, Mrs. Mould! If I was Mr. Mould, I should be jealous of you, ma'am; and I'm sure, if I was you, I should be jealous of Mr. Mould.'

'Tut, tut! Bah, bah! Go along, Mrs. Gamp!' cried the delighted undertaker.

'As to the young ladies,' said Mrs. Gamp, dropping a curtsey, 'bless their sweet looks—how they can ever reconsize it with their duties to be so grown up with such young parents, it an't for sech as me to give a guess at.'

'Nonsense, nonsense. Be off, Mrs. Gamp!' cried Mould. But in the height of his gratification, he actually pinched Mrs. Mould, as he said it.

'I'll tell you what, my dear,' he observed, when Mrs. Gamp had at last withdrawn, and shut the door, 'that's a ve-ry shrewd woman. That's a woman whose intellect is immensely superior to her station in life. That's a woman who observes and reflects in an uncommon manner. She's the sort of woman now,' said Mould, drawing his silk handkerchief over his head again, and composing himself for a nap, 'one would almost feel disposed to bury for nothing: and do it neatly, too!'

Mrs. Mould and her daughters fully concurred in these remarks; the subject of which had by this time reached the street, where she experienced so much inconvenience from the air, that she was obliged to stand under an archway for a short time, to recover herself. Even after this precaution, she walked so unsteadily as to attract the compassionate regards of divers kind-hearted boys, who took the liveliest interest in her disorder; and in their simple language, bade her be of good cheer, for she was 'only a little screwed.'

Whatever she was, or whatever name the vocabulary of medical science would have bestowed upon her malady, Mrs. Gamp was perfectly acquainted with the way home again; and arriving at the house of Anthony Chuzzlewit & Son, lay down to rest. Remaining there until seven o'clock in the evening, and then persuading poor old Chuffey to betake himself to bed, she sallied forth upon her new engagement. First, she went to her private lodgings in Kingsgate Street, for a bundle of robes and wrappings comfortable in the night season; and then repaired to the Bull of Holborn, which she reached as the clocks were striking eight.

As she turned into the yard, she stopped; for the landlord, landlady, and head-chambermaid, were all on the threshold together, talking earnestly with a young gentleman who seemed to have just come or to be just going away. The first words that struck upon Mrs. Gamp's ear obviously bore reference to the patient; and it being expedient that all good attendants should know as much as possible about the case on which their skill is brought to bear, Mrs. Gamp listened as a matter of duty.

'No better, then?' observed the gentleman.

'Worse!' said the landlord.

'Much worse,' added the landlady.

'Oh! a deal badder,' cried the chambermaid from the background, opening her eyes very wide, and shaking her head.

'Poor fellow!' said the gentleman, 'I am sorry to hear it. The worst of it is, that I have no idea what friends or relations he has, or where they live, except that it certainly is not in London.'

The landlord looked at the landlady; the landlady looked at the landlord; and the chambermaid remarked, hysterically, 'that of all the many wague directions she had ever seen or heerd of (and they wasn't few in an hotel), *that* was the waguest.'

'The fact is, you see,' pursued the gentleman, 'as I told you yesterday when you sent to me, I really know very little about him. We were schoolfellows together; but since that time I have only met him twice. On both occasions I was in London for a boy's holiday (having come up for a week or so from Wiltshire), and lost sight of him again directly. The letter bearing my name and address which you found upon his table, and which led to your applying to me, is an answer, you will observe, to one he wrote from his house the very day he was taken ill, making an appointment with him at his own request. Here is his letter, if you wish to see it.'

The landlord read it: the landlady looked over him. The chambermaid, in the background, made out as much of it as she could, and invented the rest; believing it all from that time forth as a positive piece of evidence.

'He has very little luggage, you say?' observed the gentleman, who was no other than our old friend, John Westlock.

'Nothing but a portmanteau,' said the landlord; 'and very little in it.'

'A few pounds in his purse, though?'

'Yes. It's sealed up, and in the cash-box. I made a memorandum of the amount, which you're welcome to see.'

'Well!' said John, 'as the medical gentleman says the fever must take its course, and nothing can be done just now beyond giving him his drinks regularly and having him carefully attended to, nothing more can be said that I know of, until he is in a condition to give us some information. Can you suggest anything else?'

'N-no,' replied the landlord, 'except—'

'Except, who's to pay, I suppose?' said John.

'Why,' hesitated the landlord, 'it would be as well.'

'Quite as well,' said the landlady.

'Not forgetting to remember the servants,' said the chambermaid in a bland whisper.

'It is but reasonable, I fully admit,' said John Westlock. 'At all events, you have the stock in hand to go upon for the present; and I will readily undertake to pay the doctor and the nurses.'

'Ah!' cried Mrs. Gamp. 'A rayal gentleman.'

She groaned her admiration so audibly, that they all turned round. Mrs. Gamp felt the necessity of advancing, bundle in hand, and introducing herself.

'The night-nurse,' she observed, 'from Kingsgate Street, well beknown to Mrs. Prig, the day-nurse, and the best of creeturs. How is the poor dear gentleman, to-night? If he an't no better yet, still that is what must be expected and prepared for. It an't the fust time by a many score, ma'am,' dropping a curtsey to the landlady, 'that Mrs. Prig and me has nussed together, turn and turn about, one off, one on. We knows each other's ways, and often gives relief when others failed. Our charges is but low, sir': Mrs. Gamp addressed herself to John on this head: 'considerin' the nater of our painful dooty. If they wos made accordin' to our wishes, they would be easy paid.'

Regarding herself as having now delivered her inauguration address, Mrs. Gamp curtsied all round, and signified her wish to be conducted to the scene of her official duties. The chambermaid led her, through a variety of intricate passages, to the top of the house; and pointing at length to a solitary door at the end of a gallery, informed her that yonder was the chamber where the patient lay. That done, she hurried off with all the speed she could make.

Mrs. Gamp traversed the gallery in a great heat from having carried her large bundle up so many stairs, and tapped at the door, which was immediately opened by Mrs. Prig, bonneted and shawled and all impatience to be gone. Mrs. Prig was of the Gamp build, but not so fat; and her voice was deeper and more like a man's. She had also a beard.

'I began to think you warn't a coming!' Mrs. Prig observed, in some displeasure.

'I shall be made good to-morrow night,' said Mrs. Gamp, 'honourable. I had to go and fetch my things.' She had begun to make signs of inquiry in reference to the position of the patient and his over-hearing them—for there was a screen before the door—when Mrs. Prig settled that point easily.

'Oh!' she said aloud, 'he's quiet, but his wits is gone. It an't no matter wot you say.'

'Anythin' to tell afore you goes, my dear?' asked Mrs. Gamp, setting her bundle down inside the door, and looking affectionately at her partner.

'The pickled salmon,' Mrs. Prig replied, 'is quite delicious. I can partick'ler recommend it. Don't have nothink to say to the cold meat, for it tastes of the stable. The drinks is all good.'

Mrs. Gamp expressed herself much gratified.

'The physic and the things is on the drawers and mankleshelf,' said Mrs. Prig, cursorily. 'He took his last slime draught at seven. The easy-chair an't soft enough. You'll want his piller.'

Mrs. Gamp thanked her for these hints, and giving her a friendly good-night, held the door open until she had disappeared at the other end of the gallery. Having thus performed the hospitable duty of seeing her safely off, she shut it, locked it on the inside, took up her bundle, walked round the screen, and entered on her occupation at the sick chamber.

'A little dull, but no so bad as might be,' Mrs. Gamp remarked. 'I'm glad to see a parapidge, in case of fire, and lots of roofs and chimley-pots to walk upon.'

It will be seen from these remarks that Mrs. Gamp was looking out of window. When she had exhausted the prospect, she tried the easy-chair, which she indignantly declared was 'harder than a brick-badge.' Next she pursued her researches among the physic-bottles, glasses, jugs, and tea-cups: and when she had entirely satisfied her curiosity on all these subjects of investigation, she untied her bonnet-strings and strolled up to the bedside to take a look at the patient.

A young man—dark and not ill-looking—with long black hair, that seemed the blacker for the whiteness of the bedclothes. His eyes were partly open, and he never ceased to roll his head from side to side upon the pillow, keeping his body almost quiet. He did not utter words; but every now and then gave vent to an expression of impatience or fatigue, sometimes of surprise; and still his restless head—oh, weary, weary hour!—went to and fro without a moment's intermission.

Mrs. Gamp solaced herself with a pinch of snuff, and stood looking at him with her head inclined a little sideways, as a connoisseur might gaze upon a doubtful work of art. By degrees, a horrible remembrance of one branch of her calling took possession of the woman; and stooping down, she pinned his wandering arms against his sides, to see how he would look if laid out as a dead man. Hideous as it may appear, her fingers itched to compose his limbs in that last marble attitude.

'Ah!' said Mrs. Gamp, walking away from the bed, 'he'd make a lovely corpse.'

She now proceeded to unpack her bundle; lighted a candle with the aid of a fire-box on the drawers; filled a small kettle, as a preliminary to refreshing herself with a cup of tea in the course of the night; laid what she called 'a little bit of fire,' for the same philanthropic purpose; and also set forth a small tea-board, that nothing might be wanting for her comfortable enjoyment. These preparations occupied so long, that when they were brought to a conclusion it was high time to think about supper; so she rang the bell and ordered it.

'I think, young woman,' said Mrs. Gamp to the assistant-chamber-maid, in a tone expressive of weakness, 'that I could pick a little bit of pickled salmon, with a nice little sprig of fennel, and a sprinkling of white pepper. I takes new bread, my dear, with jest a little pat of fresh butter, and a mossel of cheese. In case there should be such a thing as a cowcumber in the 'ouse, will you be so kind as bring it, for I'm rather partial to 'em, and they does a world of good in a sick room. If they draws the Brighton Old Tipper here, I takes *that* ale at night, my love; it bein' considered wakeful by the doctors. And whatever you do, young woman, don't bring more than a shilling's-worth of gin-and-water warm when I rings the bell a second time: for that is always my allowance, and I never takes a drop beyond!'

Having preferred these moderate requests, Mrs. Gamp observed that she would stand at the door until the order was executed, to the end that the patient might not be disturbed by her opening it a second time; and therefore she would thank the young woman to 'look sharp.'

A tray was brought with everything upon it, even to the cucumber; and Mrs. Gamp accordingly sat down to eat and drink in high good-humour. The extent to which she availed herself of the vinegar, and supped up that refreshing fluid with the blade of her knife, can scarcely be expressed in narrative.

'Ah!' sighed Mrs. Gamp, as she meditated over the warm shilling's-worth, 'what a blessed thing it is—living in a wale—to be contented! What a blessed thing it is to make sick people happy in their beds, and never mind one's-self as long as one can do a service! I don't believe a finer cowcumber was ever grow'd. I'm sure I never see one.'

She moralised in the same vein until her glass was empty, and then administered the patient's medicine, by the simple process of clutching his windpipe to make him gasp, and immediately pouring it down his throat.

'I a'most forgot the piller, I declare!' said Mrs. Gamp, drawing it away. 'There! Now he's comfortable as he can be, *I*'m sure! I must try to make myself as much so as I can.'

With this view, she went about the construction of an extempo-raneous bed in the easy-chair, with the addition of the next easy one for her feet. Having formed the best couch that the circumstances admitted of, she took out of her bundle a yellow night-cap, of prodigious size, in shape resembling a cabbage; which article of dress she fixed and tied on with the utmost care, previously divesting herself of a row of bald old curls that could scarcely be called false, they were so very innocent of anything approaching to deception. From the same repository she brought forth a night-jacket, in which she also attired herself. Finally, she produced a watchman's coat, which she tied around her neck by the sleeves, so that she became two people; and looked, behind, as if she were in the act of being embraced by one of the old patrol.

All these arrangements made, she lighted the rush-light, coiled herself up on her couch, and went to sleep. Ghostly and dark the room became, and full of lowering shadows. The distant noises in the streets were gradually hushed; the house was quiet as a sepulchre; the dead of night was coffined in the silent city.

Oh, weary, weary hour! Oh, haggard mind, groping darkly through the past; incapable of detaching itself from the miserable present; dragging its heavy chain of care through imaginary feasts and revels, and scenes of awful pomp; seking but a moment's rest among the long-forgotten haunts of childhood, and the resorts of yesterday; and dimly finding fear and horror everywhere! Oh, weary, weary hour! What were the wanderings of Cain, to these?

Still, without a moment's interval, the burning head tossed to and fro. Still, from time to time, fatigue, impatience, suffering, and surprise, found utterance upon that rack, and plainly too, though never once in words. At length, in the solemn hour of midnight, he began to talk; waiting awfully for answers sometimes; as though invisible companions were about his bed; and so replying to their speech and questioning again.

Mrs. Gamp awoke, and sat up in her bed: presenting on the wall the shadow of a gigantic night constable, struggling with a prisoner.

'Come! Hold your tongue!' she cried, in sharp reproof. 'Don't make none of that noise here.'

There was no alteration in the face, or in the incessant motion of the head, but he talked on wildly.

'Ah!' said Mrs. Gamp, coming out of the chair with an impatient shiver; 'I thought I was a sleepin' too pleasant to last! The devil's in the night, I think, it's turned so chilly!'

Don't drink so much!' cried the sick man. 'You'll ruin us all. Don't you see how the fountain sinks? Look at the mark where the sparkling water was just now!'

'Sparkling water, indeed!' said Mrs. Gamp. 'I'll have a sparkling cup o' tea, I think. I wish you'd hold your noise!'

He burst into a laugh, which, being prolonged, fell off into a dismal wail. Checking himself, with fierce inconstancy he began to count, fast.

'One—two—three—four—five—six.'

' "One, two, buckle my shoe," ' said Mrs. Gamp, who was now on her knees, lighting the fire,' "three, four, shut the door,"—I wish you'd shut your mouth, young man—"five, six, picking up sticks." If I'd got a few handy, I should have the kettle biling all the sooner.'

Awaiting this desirable consummation, she sat down so close to the fender (which was a high one) that her nose rested upon it; and for some time she drowsily amused herself by sliding that feature backwards and forwards along the brass top, as far as she could, without changing her position to do it. She maintained, all the while, a running commentary upon the wanderings of the man in bed.

'That makes five hundred and twenty-one men, all dressed alike, and with the same distortion on their faces, that have passed in at the window, and out at the door,' he cried, anxiously. 'Look there! Five hundred and twenty-two—twenty-three—twenty-four. Do you see them?'

'Ah! I see 'em' said Mrs. Gamp; 'all the whole kit of 'em numbered like hackney-coaches, ain't they?'

'Touch me! Let me be sure of this. Touch me!'

'You'll take your next draught when I've made the kettle bile,' retorted Mrs. Gamp, composedly, 'and you'll be touched then. You'll be touched up, too, if you don't take it quiet.'

'Five hundred and twenty-eight, five hundred and twenty-nine, five hundred and thirty,—look here!'

'What's the matter now?' said Mrs. Gamp.

'They're coming four abreast, each man with his arm entwined in the next man's, and his hand upon his shoulder. What's that upon the arm of every man, and on the flag?'

'Spiders, p'raps,' said Mrs. Gamp.

'Crape! Black crape! Good God! why do they wear it outside?'

'Would you have 'em carry black crape in their insides?' Mrs. Gamp retorted. 'Hold your noise, hold your noise.'

The fire beginning by this time to impart a grateful warmth, Mrs. Gamp became silent; gradually rubbed her nose more and more slowly along the top of the fender; and fell into a heavy doze. She was awakened by the room ringing (as she fancied) with a name she knew—

'Chuzzlewit!'

The sound was so distinct and so real, and so full of agonised en-
treaty, that Mrs. Gamp jumped up in terror, and ran to the door.
She expected to find the passage filled with people, come to tell her
that the house in the City had taken fire. But the place was empty:
not a soul was there. She opened the window, and looked out. Dark,
dull, dingy, and desolate house-tops. As she passed to her seat again,
she glanced at the patient. Just the same; but silent. Mrs. Gamp was
so warm now, that she threw off the watchman's coat and fanned
herself.

'It seemed to make the wery bottles ring,' she said. 'What could
I have been a dreaming of? That dratted Chuffey, I'll be bound.'

The supposition was probable enough. At any rate, a pinch of
snuff, and the song of the steaming kettle, quite restored the tone of
Mrs. Gamp's nerves, which were none of the weakest. She brewed her
tea; made some buttered toast; and sat down at the tea-board, with
her face to the fire.

When once again, in a tone more terrible than that which had
vibrated in her slumbering ear, these words were shrieked out—

'Chuzzlewit! Jonas! No!'

Mrs. Gamp dropped the cup she was in the act of raising to her
lips, and turned round with a start that made her little tea-board
leap. The cry had come from the bed.

It was bright morning the next time Mrs. Gamp looked out of
the window, and the sun was rising cheerfully. Lighter and lighter
grew the sky, and noisier the streets; and high into the summer air
uprose the smoke of newly-kindled fires, until the busy day was broad-
awake.

Mrs. Prig relieved punctually, having passed a good night at her
other patient's. Mr. Westlock came at the same time, but he was not
admitted, the disorder being infectious. The doctor came too. The
doctor shook his head. It was all he could do, under the circumstances,
and he did it well.

'What sort of a night, nurse?'

'Restless, sir,' said Mrs. Gamp.

'Talk much?'

'Middling, sir,' said Mrs. Gamp.

'Nothing to the purpose, I suppose?'

'Oh bless you no, sir. Only jargon.'

'Well!' said the doctor, 'we must keep him quiet; keep the room
cool; give him his draughts regularly; and see that he's carefully looked
to. That's all!'

'And as long as Mrs. Prig and me waits upon him, sir, no fear of that,' said Mrs. Gamp.

'I suppose,' observed Mrs. Prig, when they had curtsied the doctor out: 'there's nothin' new?'

'Nothin' at all, my dear,' said Mrs. Gamp. 'He's rather wearin' in his talk from making up a lot of names; elseways you needn't mind him.'

'Oh, I shan't mind him,' Mrs. Prig returned. 'I have somethin' else to think of.'

'I pays my debts to-night, you know, my dear, and comes afore my time,' said Mrs. Gamp. 'But, Betsey Prig': speaking with great feeling, and laying her hand upon her arm: 'try the cowcumbers, God bless you!" . . .

In the previous selection Charles Dickens depicts the much-accepted stereotype of the "typical" nineteenth century nurse. Exaggerated as the familiar figure of Mrs. Gamp may be, the nurse was nonetheless a member of the servant class on a level with the scullery maid which explains the opposition of the Nightingale family to Florence's interest in the occupation. The following essay, "Cassandra", written by Florence Nightingale herself in 1852, contains the bitter and impassioned comments upon the position of women in Victorian England as she herself experienced it. While attempting to break through the artificiality that surrounded Victorian women, the commentary nonetheless also reflects Miss Nightingale's frustration and even suffering because of the family's rejection of her career choice.

FLORENCE NIGHTINGALE (1820-1910)

"Cassandra": the Plight of Women in Early Victorian England*

I

"The voice of one crying in the" crowd, "Prepare ye the way of the Lord."

One often comes to be thus wandering alone in the bitterness of life without. It might be that such as one might be tempted to seek an escape in the hope of a more congenial sphere. Yet, perhaps, if prematurely we dismiss ourselves from this world, all may even have to be suffered through again—the premature birth may not contribute

*This fragment "Cassandra", ends the second volume entitled "Practical Deductions", of Miss Nightingale's unpublished book *Suggestions for Thought to Searchers After Religious Truth*. The book was written in 1852, when she was thirty two years old, revised and finally put together in 1859, after her return from the Crimea. In that year she had it printed privately, but on the advice of John Stuart Mill, Benjamin Jowett and many other friends it was not published. It was published for the first time in 1928 as Appendix I in Mrs. Ray Strachey's *History of the Women's Movement in Great Britain* by permission of representatives of Miss Nightingale's family and executors.

to the production of another being, which must be begun again from
the beginning.

Such as one longs to replunge into the happy unconscious sleep
of the rest of the race! they slumber in one another's arms—they are
not yet awake. To them evil and suffering are not, for they are not
conscious of evil. While one alone, awake and prematurely alive to it,
must wander out in silence and solitude—such as one has awakened too
early, has risen up too soon, has rejected the companionship of the
race, unlinked to any human being. Such as one sees the evil they do
not see, and yet has no power to discover the remedy for it.

Why have women passion, intellect, moral activity—these three
—and a place in society where no one of the three can be exercised?
Men say that God punishes for complaining. No, but men are angry
with misery. They are irritated with women for not being happy. They
take it as a personal offence. To God alone may women complain without insulting Him!

And women, who are afraid, while in words they acknowledge
that God's work is good, to say. Thy will be *not* done (declaring another
order of society from that which He has made), go about maudling to
each other and teaching to their daughters that "women have no passions." In the conventional society, which men have made for women,
and women have accepted, they *must* have none, they *must* act the
farce of hypocrisy, the lie that they are without passion—and therefore
what else can they say to their daughters, without giving the lie to
themselves?

Suffering, sad "female humanity!" What are these feelings which
they are taught to consider as disgraceful, to deny to themselves? What
form do the Chinese feet assume when denied their proper development? If the young girls of the "higher classes," who never commit a
false step, whose justly earned reputations were never sullied even by
the stain which the fruit of mere "knowledge of good and evil" leaves
behind, were to speak, and say what are their thoughts employed upon,
their *thoughts*, which alone are free, what would they say?

That, with the phantom companion of their fancy, they talk (not
love, they are too innocent, too pure, too full of genius and imagination
for that, but) they talk, in fancy, of that which interests them most;
they seek a companion for their every thought; the companion they
find not in reality they seek in fancy, or, if not that, if not absorbed in
endless conversations, they see themselves engaged with him in stirring
events, circumstances which call out the interest wanting to them. Yes,
fathers, mothers, you who see your daughter proudly rejecting all
semblance of flirtation, primly engaged in the duties of the breakfast

table, you little think how her fancy compensates itself by endless interviews and sympathies (sympathies either for ideas or events) with the fancy's companion of the hour! And you say, "She is not susceptible. Women have no passion." Mothers, who cradle yourselves in visions about the domestic hearth, how many of your sons and daughters are *there*, do you think, while sitting round under your complacent eye? Were you there yourself during your own (now forgotten) girlhood?

What are the thoughts of these young girls while one is singing Schubert, another is reading the *Review*, and a third is busy embroidering? Is not one fancying herself the nurse of some new friend in sickness; another engaging in romantic dangers with him, such as call out the character and afford more food for sympathy than the monotonous events of domestic society; another undergoing unheard-of trials under the observation of someone whom she has chosen as the companion of her dream; another having a loving and loved companion in the life she is living, which many do not want to change?

And is not this all most natural, inevitable? Are they, who are too much ashamed of it to confess it even to themselves, to be blamed for that which cannot be otherwise, the causes of which stare one in the face, *if one's eyes were not closed?* Many struggle against this as a "snare." No Trappist ascetic watches or fasts more in the body than these do in the soul! They understand the discipline of the Thebaid—the life-long agonies to which those strong moral Mohicans subjected themselves. How cordially they could do the same, in order to escape the worse torture of wandering "vain imaginations." By the laws of God for moral well-being are not thus to be obeyed. We fast mentally, scourge ourselves morally, use the intellectual hair-shirt, in order to subdue that perpetual day-dreaming, which is so dangerous! We resolve "this day month I will be free from it"; twice a day with prayer and written record of the times when we have indulged in it, we endeavour to combat it. Never, with the slightest success. By mortifying vanity we do ourselves no good. It is the want of interest in our life which produces it; by filling up that want of interest in our life we can alone remedy it. And, did we even see this, how can we make the difference? How obtain the interest which society declares *she* does not want, and we cannot want? . . .

II

"Yet I would spare no pang,
Would wish no torture less,
The more that anguish racks,
The earlier it will bless."

Give use back our suffering, we cry to Heaven in our hearts—
suffering rather than indifferentism; for out of nothing comes nothing.
But out of suffering may come the cure. Better have pain than paralysis!
A hundred struggle and drown in the breakers. One discovers the new
world. But rather, ten times rather, die in the surf, heralding the way to
that new world, than stand idly on the shore!

Passion, intellect, moral activity—these three have never been
satisfied in a woman. In this cold and oppressive conventional atmosphere, they cannot be satisfied. To say more on this subject would
be to enter into the whole history of society, of the present state of
civilisation.

Look at that lizard—"It is not hot," he says, "I like it. The atmosphere which enervates you is life to me." The state of society which
some complain of makes others happy. Why should these complain to
those? *They* do not suffer. *They* would not understand it, any more
than that lizard would comprehend the sufferings of a Shetland sheep.

The progressive world is necessarily divided into two classes—
those who take the best of what there is and enjoy it—those who wish
for something better and try to create it. Without these two classes the
world would be badly off. They are the very conditions of progress,
both the one and the other. Were there none who were discontented
with what they have, the world would never reach anything better.
And, through the other class, which is constantly taking the best of
what the first is creating for them, a balance is secured, and that which
is conquered is held fast. But with neither class must we quarrel for not
possessing the privileges of the other. The laws of the nature of each
make it impossible.

Is discontent a privilege?

Yes, it is a privilege for you to suffer for your race—a privilege not
reserved to the Redeemer, and the martyrs alone, but one enjoyed by
numbers in every age.

The common-place life of thousands; and in that is its only interest—its only merit as a history; viz. that it *is* the type of common sufferings—the story of one who has not the courage to resist nor to submit
to the civilisation of her time—is this.

Poetry and imagination begin life. A child will fall on its knees on
the gravel walk at the sight of a pink hawthorn in full flower, when it is
by itself, to praise God for it.

Then comes intellect. It wishes to satisfy the wants which intellect
creates for it. But there is a physical, not moral, impossibility of supplying the wants of the intellect in the state of civilisation at which we

have arrived. The stimulus, the training, the time, are all three wanting to us; or, in other words, the means and inducements are not there.

Look at the poor lives we lead. It is a wonder that we are so good as we are, not that we are so bad. In looking round we are struck with the power of the organisations we see, not with their want of power. Now and then, it is true, we are conscious that *there* is an inferior organisation, but, in general, just the contrary. Mrs. A. has the imagination, the poetry of a Murillo, and has sufficient power of execution to show that she might have had a great deal more. Why is she not a Murillo? From a material difficulty, not a mental one. If she has a knife and fork in her hands for three hours of the day, she cannot have a pencil or brush. Dinner is the great sacred ceremony of this day, the great sacrament. To be absent from dinner is equivalent to being ill. Nothing else will excuse us from it. Bodily incapacity is the only apology valid. If she has a pen and ink in her hands during other three hours, writing answers for the penny post, again, she cannot have her pencil, and so *ad infinitum* through life. People have no type before them in their lives, neither fathers nor mothers, nor the children themselves. They look at things in detail. They say, "It is very desirable that A., my daughter, should go to such a party, should know such a lady, should sit by such a person." It is true. But what standard have they before them of the nature and destination of man? The very words are rejected as pedantic. But might they not, at least, have a type in their minds that such an one might be a discoverer through her intellect, such another through her art, a third through her moral power?

Women often try one branch of intellect after another in their youth, *e.g.* mathematics. But that, least of all is compatible with the life of "society." It is impossible to follow up anything systematically. Women often long to enter some man's profession where they would find direction, competition (or rather opportunity of measuring the intellect with others) and, above all, time.

In those wise institutions, mixed as they are with many follies, which will last as long as the human race lasts, because they are adapted to the wants of the human race; those institutions which we call monasteries, and which, embracing much that is contrary to the laws of nature, are yet better adapted to the union of the life of action and that of thought than any other mode of life with which we are acquainted; in many such, four and a half hours, at least, are daily set aside for thought, rules are given for thought, training and opportunity afforded. Among us there is *no* time appointed for this purpose, and the difficulty is that, in our social life, we must be always doubtful whether we ought not to be with somebody else or be doing something else.

Are men better off than women in this?

If one calls upon a friend in London and sees her son in the drawing-room, it strikes one as odd to find a young man sitting idle in his mother's drawing-room in the morning. For men, who are seen much in those haunts, there is no end of the epithets we have: "knights of the carpet," "drawing-room heroes," "ladies' men." But suppose we were to see a number of men in the morning sitting round a table in the drawing-room, looking at prints, doing worsted work, and reading little books, how we should laugh! A member of the House of Commons was once known to do worsted work. Of another man was said, "His only fault is that he is too good; he drives out with his mother every day in the carriage, and if he is asked anywhere he answers that he must dine with his mother, but, if she can spare him, he will come in to tea, and does not come."

Now, why is it more ridiculous for a man than for a woman to do worsted work and drive out every day in the carriage? Why should we laugh if we were to see a parcel of men sitting round a drawing-room table in the morning, and think it all right if they were women?

Is man's time more valuable than woman's? or is the difference between man and woman this, that woman has confessedly nothing to do?

Women are never supposed to have any occupation of sufficient importance *not* to be interrupted, except "suckling their fools"; and women themselves have accepted this, have written books to support it, and have trained themselves so as to consider whatever they do as *not* of such value to the world or to others, but that they can throw it up at the first "claim of social life." They have accustomed themselves to consider intellectual occupation as a merely selfish amusement, which it is their "duty" to give up for every trifler more selfish than themselves.

A young man (who was afterwards useful and known in his day and generation) when busy reading and sent for by his proud mother to shine in some morning visit, came; but, after it was over, he said, "Now, remember, this is not to happen again. I came that you might not think me sulky, but I shall not come again." But for a young woman to send such a message to her mother and sisters, how impertinent it would be! A woman of great administrative powers said that she never undertook anything which she "could not throw by at once, if necessary."

How do we explain then the many cases of women who have distinguished themselves in classics, mathematics, even in politics?

Widowhood, ill-health, or want of bread, these three explanations or excuses are supposed to justify a woman taking up an occupation. In some cases, no doubt, an indomitable force of character will suffice without any of these three, but such are rare.

But see how society fritters away the intellects of those comitted to her charge! It is said that society is necessary to sharpen the intellect. But what do we seek society for? It does sharpen the intellect, because it is a kind of *tour-de-force* to say something at a pinch,—unprepared and uninterested with any subject, to improvise something under difficulties. But what "go we out for to seek"? To take the chance of some one having something to say which we want to hear? or of finding something to say which *they* want to hear? You have a little to say, but not much. You often make a stipulation with someone else, "Come in ten minutes, for I shall not be able to find enough to spin out long than that." You are not to talk of anything very interesting, for the essence of society is to prevent any long conversations and all tête-à-têtes. *Glissez, n'appuyez pas* is its very motto. The praise of a good *maitresse de maison* consists in this, that she allows no one person to be too much absorbed in, or too long about, a conversation. She always recalls them to their "duty." People do not go into the company of their fellow-creatures for what would seem a very sufficient reason, namely, that they have something to say to them, or something that they want to hear from them; but in the vague hope that they find something to say.

Then as to solitary opportunities. Women never have an half-hour in all their lives (excepting before or after anybody is up in the house) that they can call their own, without fear of offending or of hurting someone. Why do people sit up so late, or, more rarely, get up so early? Not because the day is not long enough, but because they have "no time in the day to themselves."

If we do attempt to do anything in company, what is the system of literary exercise which we pursue? Everybody reads aloud out of their own book or newspaper—or, every five minutes, something is said. And what is it to be "read aloud to"? The most miserable exercise of the human intellect. Or rather, is it any exercise at all? It is like lying on one's back, with one's hands tied and having liquid poured down one's throat. Worse than that, because suffocation would immediately ensue and put a stop to this operation. But no suffocation would stop the other.

So much for the satisfaction of the intellect. Yet for a married woman in society, it is even worse. A married woman was heard to wish

that she could break a limb that she might have a little time to herself.
Many take advantage of the fear of "infection" to do the same.

It is a thing *so* accepted among women that they have nothing to
do, that one woman has not the least scruple in saying to another, "I
will come and spend the morning with you." And you would be thought
quite surly and absurd, if you were to refuse it on the plea of occupation. Nay, it is thought a mark of amiability and affection, if you are
"on such terms" that you can "come in" "any morning you please."

In a country house, if there is a large party of young people, "You
will spend the morning with us," they say to the neighbours, "we will
drive together in the afternoon," "to-morrow we will make an expedition, and we will spend the evening together." And this is thought
friendly and spending time in a pleasant manner. So women play
through life. Yet time is the most valuable of all things. If they had
come every morning and afternoon and robbed us of half-a-crown we
should have had redress from the police. But it is laid down, that our
time is of no value. If you offer a morning visit to a professional man,
and say, "I will just stay an hour with you, if you will allow me, till so
and so comes back to fetch me"; it costs him the earnings of an hour,
and therefore he has a right to complain. But women have no right,
because it is "*only* their time."

Women have no means given them, whereby they *can* resist the
"claims of social life." They are taught from their infancy upwards
that it is a wrong, ill-tempered, and a misunderstanding of "woman's
mission" (with a great M) if they do not allow themselves *willingly* to
be interrupted at all hours. If a woman has once put in a claim to be
treated as a man by some work of science or art or literature, which
she can *show* as the "fruit of her leisure," then she will be considered
justified in *having* leisure (hardly, perhaps, even then). But if not, not.
If she has nothing to show, she must resign herself to her fate.

. . . Women often strive to live by intellect. The clear, brilliant,
sharp radiance of intellect's moonlight rising upon such an expanse of
snow is dreary, it is true, but some love its solemn desolation, its
silence, its solitude—if they are but *allowed* to live in it; if they are not
perpetually baulked or disappointed. But a woman cannot live in the
light of intellect. Society forbids it. Those conventional frivolities,
which are called her "duties," forbid it. Her "domestic duties" high-
sounding words, which, for the most part, are bad habits (which she
has not the courage to enfranchise herself from, the strength to break
through) forbid it. What are these duties (or bad habits)?—Answering a
multitude of letters which lead to nothing, from her so-called friends,

keeping herself up to the level of the world that she may furnish her quota of amusement at the breakfast-table; driving out her company in the carriage. And all these things are exacted from her by her family which, if she is good and affectionate, will have more influence with her than the world.

What wonder, if, wearied out, sick at heart with hope deferred, the springs of will broken, not seeing clearly *where* her duty lies, she abandons intellect as a vocation and takes it only, as we use the moon, by glimpses through her tight-closed window shutters?

The family? It is too narrow a field for the development of an immortal spirit, be that spirit male or female. The chances are a thousand to one that, in that small sphere, the task for which that immortal spirit is destined by the qualities and the gifts which its Creator has placed within it, will not be found.

The family uses people, *not* for what they are, nor for what they are intended to be, but for what it wants them for—its own uses. It thinks of them not as what God has made them, but as the something which it has arranged that they shall be. If it wants someone to sit in the drawing-room, *that* someone is supplied by the family, though that member may be destined for science, or for education, or for active superintendence by God, *i.e.* by the gifts within.

This system dooms some minds to incurable infancy, others to silent misery.

And family boasts that it has performed its mission well, in as far as it has enabled the individual to say, "I have *no* peculiar work, nothing but what the moment brings me, nothing that I cannot throw up at once at anybody's claim"; in as far, that is, as it has *destroyed* the individual life. And the individual thinks that a great victory has been accomplished, when, at last, she is able to say that she has "no personal desires or plans." What is this but throwing the gifts of God aside as worthless, and substituting for them those of the world?

Marriage is the only chance (and it is but a chance) offered to women for escape from this death; and how eagerly and how ignorantly it is embraced!

At present we live to impede each other's satisfactions; competition, domestic life, society, what is it all but this? We go somewhere where we are not wanted and where we don't want to go. What else is conventional life? *Passivity* when we want to be active. So many hours spent every day in passively going what conventional life tells us, when we would so gladly be at work.

And is it a wonder that all individual life is extinguished?

Women dream of a great sphere of steady, not sketchy bene-volence, of moral activity, for which they would fain be trained and fitted, instead of working in the dark, neither knowing nor registering whither their steps lead, whether farther from or nearer to the aim ...

... Women long for an education to teach them *to teach*, to teach them the laws of the human mind and how to apply them—and knowing how imperfect, in the present state of the world, such an education must be, they long for experience, not patch-work experience, but experience followed up and systematised, to enable them to know what they are about and *where* they are "casting their bread," and whether it is "*bread*" or a stone.

How should we learn a language if we were to give it an hour a week? A fortnight's steady application would make more way in it than a year of such patch-work. A "lady" can hardly go to "her school" two days running. She cannot leave the breakfast-table—or she must be fulfilling some little frivolous "duty," which others ought not to exact, or which might just as well be done some other time.

Dreaming always—never accomplishing; thus women live—too much ashamed of their dreams, which they think "romantic," to tell them where they will be laughed at, even if not considered wrong.

With greater strength of purpose they might accomplish some-thing. But if they were strong, all of them, they would not need to have their story told, for all the world would read it in the mission they have fulfilled. It is for common-place, every-day characters that we tell our tale—because it is the sample of hundreds of lives (or rather deaths) of persons who cannot fight with society, or who, unsupported by the sympathies about them, give up their own destiny as not worth the fierce and continued struggle necessary to accomplish it. *One* struggle they *could* make and be free (and, in the Church of Rome, many, many, unallured by any other motive, make this one struggle to enter a convent); but the perpetual series of petty spars, with dis-couragements between, and doubts as to whether they are right—these wear out the very life necessary to make them.

If a man were to follow up his profession or occupation at odd times, how would he do it? Would he become skilful in that profession? It is acknowledged by women themselves that they are inferior in every occupation to men. Is it wonderful? *They* do *everything* at "odd times."

And if a woman's music and drawing are only used by her as an amusement (*a pass-time*, as it is called), is it wonderful that she tires of them, that she becomes disgusted with them?

In every dream of the life of intelligence or that of activity, took to hers very kindly; insomuch, that setting aside her natural predilections as a woman, she went to a lying-in or a laying-out with equal zest and relish. . . .

. . . 'Tell Mrs. Gamp to come upstairs,' said Mould. 'Now, Mrs. Gamp, what's *your* news?'

The lady in question was by this time in the door-way, curtseying to Mrs. Mould. At the same moment a peculiar fragrance was borne upon the breeze, as if a passing fairy had hiccoughed, and had previously been to a wine-vault.

Mrs. Gamp made no response to Mr. Mould, but curtsied to Mrs. Mould again, and held up her hands and eyes, as in a devout thanksgiving that she looked so well. She was neatly, but not gaudily attired, in the weeds she had worn when Mr. Pecksniff had the pleasure of making her acquaintance; and was perhaps the turning of a scale more snuffy.

'There are some happy creeturs,' Mrs. Gamp observed, 'as time runs back-ards with, and you are one, Mrs. Mould; not that he need do nothing except use you in his most owldacious way for years to come, I'm sure; for young you are and will be. I says to Mrs. Harris,' Mrs. Gamp continued, 'only t' other day; the last Monday evening fortnight as ever dawned upon this Piljian's Projiss of a mortal wale; I says to Mrs. Harris when she says to me, "Years and our trials, Mrs. Gamp, sets marks upon us all."—"Say not the words, Mrs. Harris, if you and me is to be continual friends, for sech is not the case. Mrs. Mould," I says, making so free, I will confess, as use the name,' (she curtsied here), ' "is one of them that goes agen the observation straight; and never, Mrs. Harris, whilst I've a drop of breath to draw, will I set by, and not stand up, don't think it."—"I ast your pardon, ma'am," says Mrs. Harris, "and I humbly grant your grace; for if ever a woman lived as would see her feller-creeturs into fits to serve her friends, well do I know that woman's name is Sairey Gamp." '

At this point she was fain to stop for breath; and advantage may be taken of the circumstance, to state that a fearful mystery surrounded this lady of the name of Harris, whom no one in the circle of Mrs. Gamp's acquaintance had ever seen; neither did any human being know her place of residence, though Mrs. Gamp appeared on her own showing to be in constant communication with her. There were conflicting rumours on the subject; but the prevalent opinion was that she was a phantom of Mrs. Gamp's brain—as Messrs. Doe and Roe are fictions of the law—created for the express purpose of holding visionary dialogues with her on all manner of subjects, and invariably winding up with a compliment to the excellence of her nature.

by a phantom—the phantom of sympathy
—even if they do not marry. Some few sacri-
y sacrifice all other life if they accept that.
e an equality of duties and rights is accepted
by man. Behind *his* destiny woman must
only his complement. A woman dedicates
her husband; she fills up and performs the
if she has any destiny, any vocation of her
, in nine cases out of ten. Some few, like
lm, Mrs Fry, have not done so; but these are
woman has so seldom any vocation of her
signify; she has none to renounce. A man
ge: he gains a "helpmate," but a woman

ne into contact with sickness, with poverty,
practical reality of life revives them! They
vho live on opium or on novels, all their
s which lead to no action. If they see and
of action, with a full and interesting life,
t up to the occupation, occupation con-
it is the *beau-ideal* of practical, not theo-
re-tempered, their life is filled, they have
ans to do it.

young, sometimes think that an actress's
the sake of the admiration, not for the
in the morning she studies, in the evening
he has the means of testing and correcting
uming her studies in the morning, to im-
y the failures, and in the evening try the
d, true that, even after middle age, with
is no end to the progress which may be

from suicide because it is in the most
d: "I will not, I will not do as Thou
it is "no use."

eads, no food for our hearts, no food for
f we have no food for the body, how do
hears of it, how all the newspapers talk
in great capital letters, DEATH FROM
one were to put a paragraph in the
Starvation, or Death of Moral Activity

from Starvation, how people would stare, how they would laugh and wonder! One would think we had no heads nor hearts, by the total indifference of the public towards them. Our bodies are the only things of any consequence.

We have nothing to do which raises us, no food which agrees with us. We can never pursue any object for a single two hours, for we can never command any regular leisure or solitude; and in social and domestic life one is bound, under pain of being thought sulky, to make a remark every two minutes.

Men are on the side of society; they blow hot and cold; they say, "Why can't you employ yourself in society?" and then, "Why don't you talk in society?" I can pursue a connected conversation, or I can be silent; but to drop a remark, as it is called every two minutes, how wearisome it is! It is impossible to pursue the current of one's own thoughts, because one must keep oneself ever on the alert, "to say something"; and it is impossible to say what one is thinking, because the essence of a remark is not to be a thought, but an impression. With what labour women have toiled to break down all individual and independent life, in order to fit themselves for this social and domestic existence, thinking it right! And when they have killed themselves to do it, they have awakened (too late) to think it wrong . . .

. . . When shall we see a woman making a *study* of what she does? Married women cannot; for a man would think, if his wife undertook any great work with the intention of carrying it out,—of making anything but a sham of it—that she would "suckle his fools and chronicle his small beer" ! well for it,—that he would not have so good a dinner—that she would destroy, as it is called, his domestic life.

The intercourse of man and woman—how frivolous, how unworthy it is! Can we call *that* the true vocation of woman—her high career? Look round at the marriages which you know. The true marriage—that noble union, by which a man and woman become together the one perfect being—probably does not exist at present upon earth.

It is not suprising that husbands and wives seem so little part of one another. It is surprising that there is so much love as there is. For there is no food for it. What does it live upon—what nourishes it? Husbands and wives never seem to have anything to say to one another. What do they talk about? Not about any great religious, social, political questions or feelings. They talk about who shall come to dinner, who is to live in this lodge and who in that, about the improvement of the place, or when they shall go to London. If there are children, they form a common subject of some nourishment. But, even then, the case

---

arles Dickens' *Martin Chuzzlewhit* (1843) has been ught to reflect the great nineteenth century novelist is highest power (D.N.B.). This literary master's power satirical portraiture and brilliance of style were all di-ed, he tells us, to one main object, "to exhibit in a ety of aspects the commonest of all the vices; to show Selfishness propagates itself; and to what a grim t it may grow, from small beginnings"(xvi). More ifically, in this excerpt from Chapter XV, none should t that his inimitable caricatures of the pseudo-nurses Gamp and Betsy Prig as "representations of the attendants on the poor in sickness"(xvii) demonstrate atically why nursing was considered an inferior and sirable occupation.

812-1870)

Betsy Prig Prevail

woman, this Mrs. Gamp, with a husky voice had a remarkable power of turning up, and it. Having very little neck, it cost her some , if one may say so, at those to whom she sty black gown, rather the worse for snuff, correspond. In these dilapidated articles of arrayed herself, time out of mind, on such this at once expressed a decent amount of and invited the next of kin to present her an appeal so frequently successful, that the Gamp, bonnet and all, might be seen hang-, in at least a dozen of the secondhand . The face of Mrs. Gamp—the nose in and swollen, and it was difficult to enjoy conscious of a smell of spirits. Like most great eminence in their profession, she is oftenest thus,—the husband is to think of how they are to get on in life; the wife of bringing them up at home.

But any real communion between husband and wife—any descending into the depths of their being, and drawing out thence what they find and comparing it—do we ever dream of such a thing? Yes, we may dream of it during the season of "passion," but we shall not find it afterwards. We even expect it to go off, and lay our account that it will. If the husband has, by chance gone into the depths of *his* being, and found there anything unorthodox, he, oftenest, conceals it carefully from his wife,—he is afraid of "unsettling her opinions."

What is the mystery of passion, spiritually speaking? For there *is* a passion of the Spirit. *Blind* passion, as it has most truly been called, seems to come on in man without his exactly knowing why for *this* person rather than for *that*, and (whether it has been satisfied or unsatisfied) to go off again awhile, as it came, also without his knowing why.

The woman's passion is generally more lasting.

It is possible that this difference may be, because there is really more in man than in woman. There is nothing in her for him to have this intimate communion *with*. He cannot impart to her his religious beliefs, if he have any, because she would be "shocked." Religious men are and must be heretics now—for we must not pray, except in a "form" of words, made beforehand—or think of God but with a pre-arranged idea.

With the man's political ideas, if they extend beyond the merest party politics, she has no sympathy.

His social ideas, if they are "advanced," she will probably denounce without knowing why, as savouring of "socialism" (a convenient word, which covers a multitude of new ideas and offences). For woman is "by birth a Tory,"—has often been said,—by education a "Tory," we mean.

Woman has nothing but her affections,—and this makes her at once more loving and less loved.

But is it surprising that there should be so little marriage, when we think what the process is which leads to marriage?

Under the eyes of an always present mother and sisters (of whom even the most refined and intellectual cannot abstain from a jest upon the subject, who think it their *duty* to be anxious, to watch every germ and bud of it) the acquaintance begins. It is fed—upon what?— the gossip of art, musical and pictorial, the party politics of the day, the chit-chat of society, and people marry or sometimes they don't marry, discouraged by the impossibility of knowing any more of one another than this will furnish

They prefer to marry in *thought*, to hold imaginary conversations with one another in idea, rather than on such a flimsy pretext of communion, to take the chance (certainly it cannot be) of having more to say to one another in marriage.

Men and women meet now *to be idle*. Is it extraordinary that they do not know each other, and that, in their mutual ignorance, they form no surer friendships? Did they meet to *do* something together, then indeed they might form some real tie.

But as it is, *they* are not there, it is only a mask which is there— a mouth-piece of ready-made sentences about the "topics of the day"; and then people rail against men for choosing a woman "for her face"— why, what else do they see?

It is very well to say "be prudent, be careful, try to know each other." But how are you to know each other?

Unless a woman had lost all pride, how is it possible for her, under the eyes of all her family, to indulge in long exclusive conversations with a man? "Such a thing" must not take place till after her "engagement." And how is she to make an engagement, if "such a thing" has not taken place?

Besides, young women at home have so little to occupy and to interest them—they have so little reason for *not* quitting their home, that a young and independent man cannot look at a girl without giving rise to "expectations" if not on her own part, on that of her family. Happy he, if he is not said to have been "trifling with her feelings," or "disappointing her hopes!" Under these circumstances, how can a man, who has any pride or principle, become acquainted with a woman in such a manner as to *justify* them in marrying?

There are four ways in which people marry. First, accident or relationship has thrown them together in their childhood, and acquaintance has grown up naturally and unconsciously. Accordingly, in novels, it is generally cousins who marry; and *now* it seems the only natural thing—the only possible way of making any intimacy. And yet, we know that intermarriage between relations is in direct contravention of the laws of nature for the well-being of the race; witness the Quakers, the Spanish grandees, the royal races, the secluded valleys of mountainous countries, where madness, degeneration of race, defective organisation and cretinism flourish and multiply.

The second way, and by far the most general, in which people marry, is this. A woman, thoroughly uninterested at home, and having formed a slight acquaintance with some accidental person, accepts him, if he "falls in love" with her, as it is technically called, and takes the chance. Hence the vulgar expression of marriage being a lottery, which it mostly truly is, for that the *right* two should come together has as many chances against it as there are blanks in any lottery.

The third way is, that some person is found sufficiently independent, sufficiently careless of the opinions of others, or sufficiently without modesty to speculate thus: "It is worth while that I should become acquainted with so and so. I do not care what his or her opinion of me is, if, *after* having become acquainted, to do which can bear no other construction in people's eyes than a desire of marriage, I retreat." But there is this to be said, that it is doubtful whether, under their unnatural tension, which, to all susceptible characters, such a disregard of the opinions which they care for must be, a healthy or a natural feeling can grow up.

And now they are married—that is to say, two people have received the licence of man in a white surplice. But they are no more man and wife for that than Louis XIV and the Infanta of Spain, married by proxy, were man and wife. The woman who has sold herself for an establishment, in what is she superior to those we may not name?

Lastly, in a few rare, very rare cases, such as circumstances, always provided in novels, but seldom to be met with in real life, present—whether the accident of parents' neglect, or of parents' unusual skill and wisdom, or of having no parents at all, which is generally the case in novels—or by marrying out of the person's rank of life, by which the usual restraints are removed, and there is room and play left for attraction—or extraordinary events, isolation, misfortunes, which many wish for, even though their imaginations be not tainted by romance-reading; such alternatives as these give food and space for the development of character and mutual sympathies. But a girl, if she has any pride, is so ashamed of having anything she wishes to say out of the hearing of her own family, she thinks it must be something so very wrong, that it is ten to one, if she have the opportunity of saying it, that she will not.

And yet she is spending her life, perhaps, in dreaming of accidental means of unrestrained communion.

And then it is thought pretty to say that "Women have no passion." If passion is excitement in the daily social intercourse with men, women think about marriage much more than men do; it is the only event of their lives. It ought to be a sacred event, but surely not the only event of a woman's life, as it is now. Many women spend their lives in asking men to marry them, in a refined way. Yet it is true that women are seldom in love. How can they be?

How cruel are the revulsions which high-minded women suffer! There was one who loved, in connexion with great deeds, noble thoughts, devoted feelings. They met after an interval. It was at one of those crowded parties of Civilisation which we call Society. His only careless passing remark was, "The buzz to-night is like a manufactory." Yet he loved her.

V

... Women dream till they have no longer the strength to dream; those dreams against which they so struggle, so honestly, vigorously, and conscientiously, and so in vain, yet which are their life, without which they could not have lived; those dreams go at last. All their plans and visions seem vanished, and they know not where; gone, and they cannot recall them. They do not even remember them. And they are left without the food of reality or of hope.

Later in life, they neither desire nor dream, neither of activity, nor of love, nor of intellect. The last often survives the longest. They wish, if their experiences would benefit anybody, to give them to someone. But they never find an hour free in which to collect their thoughts, and so discouragement becomes ever deeper and deeper, and they less and less capable of undertaking anything.

It seems as if the female spirit of the world were mourning everlasting over blessings, not *lost*, but which she has never had, and which, in her discouragement she feels that she never will have, they are so far off.

The more complete a woman's organisation, the more she will feel it, till at last there shall arise a woman, who will resume, in her own soul, all the sufferings of her race, and that women will be the Saviour of her race.

Jesus Christ raised women above the condition of mere slaves, mere ministers to the passions of the man, raised them by His sympathy, to be Ministers of God. He have them moral activity. But the Age, the World, Humanity, must give them the means to exercise this moral activity, must give them intellectual cultivation, spheres of action.

There is perhaps no century where the woman shows so meanly as in this. Because her education seems entirely to have parted company with her vocation; there is no longer unity between the woman as inwardly developed, and as outwardly manifested.

In the last century it was not so. In the succeeding one let us hope that it will no longer be so.

But now she is like the Archangel Michael as he stands upon Saint Angelo at Rome. She has an immense provision of wings, which seem as if they would bear her over earth and heaven; but when she tries to use them, she is petrified into stone, her feet are grown into the earth, chained to the bronze pedestal.

Nothing can well be imagined more painful than the present position of woman, unless, on the one hand, she renounces all outward activity and keeps herself within the magic sphere, the bubble of her dreams; or, on the other, surrendering all aspiration, she gives herself to her real life, soul and body. For those to whom it is possible, the latter is best; for out of activity may come thought, out of mere aspiration can come nothing.

But now—when the young imagination is so high and so developed, and reality is so narrow and conventional—there is no more parallelism between life in the thought and life in the actual than between the corpse, which lies motionless in its narrow bed, and the spirit, which, in our imagination, is at large among the stars.

The ideal life is passed in noble schemes of good consecutively followed up, of devotion to a great object, of sympathy given and received for high ideas and generous feelings. The actual life is passed in sympathy given and received for a dinner, a party, a piece of furniture, a house built or a garden laid out well, in devotion to your guests—(a too real devotion, for it implies that of all your time)—in schemes of schooling for the poor, which you follow up perhaps in an odd quarter of an hour, between luncheon and driving out in the carriage—broth and dripping are included in the plan—and the rest of your time goes in ordering the dinner, hunting for a governess for your children, and sending pheasants and apples to your poorer relations. Is there anything in *this* life which can be called an Incarnation of the ideal life within? Is it a wonder that the unhappy woman should prefer to keep them entirely separate? not to take the bloom off her Ideal by mixing it up with her Actual; not to make her Actual still more unpalatable by trying to *inform* it with her Ideal? And then she is blamed, and her own sex unites against her, for not being content with the "day of small things." She is told that "trifles make the sum of human things"; they do indeed. She is contemptuously asked, "Would she abolish domestic life?" Men are afraid that their houses will not be so comfortable, that their wives will make themselves "remarkable" women, that they will make themselves distasteful to men; they write books (and very wisely) to teach themselves to dramatise "little things," to persuade themselves that "domestic life is their sphere" and to idealise the "sacred hearth." Sacred it is indeed. Sacred from the touch of their sons almost as soon as they are out of childhood—from its dulness and its tyrannous trifling *these* recoil. Sacred from the grasp of their daughters' affections upon which it has so light a hold that they seize the first opportunity of marriage, *their* only chance of emancipation. The "sacred hearth"; sacred to their husband's sleep, their sons' absence in the body of their daughters' in mind.

Oh! mothers, who talk about this hearth, how much do you know of your son's real life, how much of your daughter's imaginary one? Awake, ye women, all ye that sleep, awake! If this domestic life were so very good, would your young men wander away from it, your maidens think of something else?

The time is come when women must do something more than the "domestic hearth," which means nursing the infants, keeping a pretty house, having a good dinner and an entertaining party.

You say, "It is true, our young men see visions, and our maidens dream dreams," but what of? Does not the woman intend to marry, and have over again what she has at home? and the man ultimately too? Yes, but not the same; she *will* have the same, that is, if circumstances are not altered to prevent it; but her *ideal* is very different, though that ideal and the reality will never come together to mould each other. And it is not only the unmarried woman who dreams. The married woman also holds long imaginary conversations but too often.

VI

We live in the world, it is said, and must walk in its ways.

Was Christ called a complainer against the world? Yet all these great teachers and preachers must have had a most deep and ingrained sense, a continual feeling of the miseries and wrongs of the world. Otherwise they would not have been impelled to devote life and death to redress them. Christ, Socrates, Howard, they must have had no ear for the joys, compared to that which they had for the sorrows of the world.

They acted, however, and we complain. The great reformers of the world turn into the great misanthropists, if circumstances or organisation do not permit them to act. Christ, if He had been a woman, might have been nothing but a great complainer. Peace be with the misanthropists! They have made a step in progress; the next will make them great philanthropists; they are divided but by a line.

The next Christ will perhaps be a female Christ. But do we see one woman who looks like a female Christ? or even like "the messenger before" her "face," to go before her and prepare the hearts and minds for her?

To this will be answered that half the inmates of Bedlam begin in this way, by fancying that they are "the Christ."

People talk about imitating Christ, and imitate Him in the little trifling formal things, such as washing the feet, saying His prayer, and so on; but if anyone attempts the real imitation of Him, there are no bounds to the outcry with which the presumption of that person is condemned.

For instance, Christ was saying something to the people one day, which interested Him very much, and interested them very much; and Mary and His brothers came in the middle of it, and wanted to interrupt Him, and take Him home to dinner, very likely—(how natural that story is! does it not speak more home than any historic evidences of the Gospel's reality?), and He, instead of being angry with their interruption of Him in such an important work for some trifling thing, answers, "Who is my mother? and who are my brethren? Whosoever shall do the will of my Father which is in heaven, the same is my brother and sister and mother." But if *we* were to say that, we should be accused of "destroying the family tie, of diminishing the obligation of the home duties."

He might well say, "Heaven and earth shall pass away, but my words shall not pass away." His words will never pass away. If he had said, "Tell them that I am engaged at this moment in something very important; that the instruction of the multitude ought to go before any personal ties; that I will remember to come when I have done," no one would have been impressed by His words; but how striking is that, "Behold my mother and my brethren!"

VII

The dying woman to her mourners:—"Oh! if you knew how gladly I leave this life, how much more courage I feel to take the chance of another, than of anything I see before me in this, you would put on your wedding-clothes instead of mourning for me!"

"But," they say, "so much talent! so many gifts! such good which you might have done!"

"The world will be put back some little time by my death," she says; "you see I estimate my powers at least as highly as you can; but it is by the death which has taken place some years ago in me, not by the death which is about to take place now." And so is the world put back by the death of every one who has to sacrifice the development of his or her peculiar gifts (which were meant, not for selfish gratification, but for the improvement of that world) to conventionality.

"My people were like children playing on the shore of the eighteenth century. I was their hobby-horse, their plaything; and they drove me to and fro, dear souls! never weary of the play themselves, till I, who had grown to woman's estate and to the ideas of the nineteenth century, lay down exhausted, my mind closed to hope, my heart to strength.

"Free—free—oh! divine freedom, art thou come at last? Welcome, beautiful death!"

Let neither name nor date be placed on her grave, still less the expression of regret or of admiration; but simply the words, "I believe in God."

Who was Florence Nightingale?

Sir Edward Cook's two volume biography, *The Life of Florence Nightingale 1820-1910* (1914), is universally accepted as the work that disposed of the mythical figure and replaced it with a fully human personality. While a commissioned book, which provided him access to the invaluable and indispensable Verney-Nightingale papers, the assignment was accepted only on the condition that he could pursue the truth without opposition. The result is a human portrait which, while bringing forth her many sides, reminds us that she "was by no means a Plaster Saint." Even Lytton Strachey in his notorious 1918 sketch and Mrs. Cecil Woodham-Smith, in her James Tait Black Memorial Prize award-winning biography of 1951, both admit that their respective portraits were derived from the foundation set down by Sir Edward Cook. In this "Conclusion" to the two volumes, Cook reveals his journalistic background in incisively summarizing everything about the character of this many-sided "pioneer" that has come before it.

SIR EDWARD T. COOK (1857-1919)

The Many Sides of Florence Nightingale

. . . The character and the life described in this book had many sides; and though the essential truth consists in the blending of them all, it is necessary in the medium of recital in prose to depict first one side and then another. The artist on canvas exhibits the blended tints at one time. That is why the portrait by a great painter sometimes tells us more of a character at a glance then is gathered from volumes of written biography. But no artist painted a portrait of Miss Nightingale in her prime, and I must do as best I may with my blotching prose in an endeavour to collect into some general impression what has been told in these volumes. I begin with recalling some of the stronger traits; they will presently be softened when I turn to other sides of the character which has been illustrated in this Memoir.

Florence Nightingale was by no means a Plaster Saint. She was a woman of strong passions—not over-given to praise, not quick to forgive; somewhat prone to be censorious, not apt to forget. She was not only a gentle angel of compassion; she was more a logician than a sentimentalist;

she knew that to do good work requires a hard head as well as a soft heart. It was said by Miss Nightingale of a certain great lady that "with the utmost kindness and benevolent intentions she is in consequence of want of practical habits of business nothing but good and bustling, a time-waster and an impediment." Miss Nightingale knew hardly any fault which seemed worse to her in a man than to be unbusiness-like; in a woman, than to be "only enthusiastic." She found no use for "angels without hands." She was essentially a "man of facts" and a "man of action." She had an equal contempt for those who act without knowledge, and for those whose knowledge leads to no useful action. She was herself laborious of detail and scrupulously careful of her premises. "Though I write positively," she once said, "I do not think positively." She weighed every consideration; she sought much competent advice; but when once her decision was taken, she was resolute and masterful—not lightly turned from her course, impatient of delay, not very tolerant of opposition.

Something of this spirit appears in her view of friendship and in the conduct of her affections. Men and women are placed in the world in order, she thought, to work for the betterment of the human race, and their work should be the supreme consideration. Mr. Jowett said of Miss Nightingale that she was the only woman he had ever known who put public duty before private. Whosoever did the will of the Father, the same was her brother, and sister, and mother. "*The* thing wanted in England," she wrote to Madame Mohl (April 30, 1868), "to raise women (and to raise men too) is: these friendships without love between men and women. And if between married men and married women all the better. . . . I think a woman who cares for a man because of his convictions, and who ceases to care for him if he alters those convictions, is worthy of the highest reverence. The novels—all novels, the best—which represent women as in love with men without any reason at all, and ready to leave their highest occupations for love—are to me utterly wearisome—as wearisome as a juggler's trick—or Table-turning—or Spiritual rapping, when the spirit says Aw! and that is so sublime that all the women are subjugated. Madame Récamier's going to Rome when M. de Chateaubriand was made Minister is exactly to me as a soldier deserting on the eve of a battle." The occasion of this letter was some gossip of the day about a great lady whose friendship with a politician was supposed to have cooled owing to some intellectual or political disagreement. "I have the greatest reverence for —— ; and I think hers was one of the best friendships that ever was—and for the oddest reason—what do you think?—Because she has broken it." What she said about Chateaubriand reflected, from a different point of view, something that Mr. Jowett had written to her in the previous year. "I am not at all tired," he had said (Sept. 1867), "of hearing about Lord Herbert. That was one of the best friendships which there ever was upon earth. Shall I tell you why I say this? Because you were willing to have gone to India in 1857." Devotion to a common purpose in active life and equal zeal in the co-operative prosecution of it: these were the conditions which Miss Nightingale required in friendship. They were realized the most fully in the case of five years of her friendship with Sidney Herbert—a period of which she used to speak, accordingly, as her "heaven upon earth." It was the work with him, more than the charm of his conversation and manner (though he had both and though she was susceptible to both), that was the essence of her pleasure. She had as little taste for conversation as for knowledge that led nowhither. "There is nothing so fatiguing," she said, "as a companion who is always *effleurant* the deepest subjects—never going below the surface; as a person who is always inquiring and never coming to any solution or decision. I don't know whether Hamlet was mad. But certainly he would have driven me mad."

The same positive and purposeful spirit, attuned rather to the intellectual and active sides of human nature than to the emotional, coloured Miss Nightingale's preferences in literature—as in this letter to Madame Mohl (May 20, 1868): " 'What does it pruv?' said the old Scotchwoman of *Paradise Lost*, and was abused for saying it. I say the same thing. *Paradise Lost* pruvs nothing. *Samson Agonistes* pruvs a great deal. Tennyson never pruvs anything. Browning's *Paracelsus* pruvs something. Shakespeare, in whatever he writes—in the deepest, highest tragedies, like 'King Lear' or 'Hamlet'—pruvs everything and does most explain the ordinary life of every one of us." She was a great reader, but she preferred the literature of fact to that of imagination. "Wondering," she said, "is like yawning, and leaves the same sensation behind it, and should never be allowed except when people are very much exhausted."

There followed from all this a certain severity in Miss Nightingale's dealings with her friends; a certain inability to show tolerance or understanding for other points of view than her own. There was a lady, once a fellow-worker, who accused Miss Nightingale roundly of having "no idea of friendship." The accusation was not true, but one can see what the lady meant. Miss Nightingale was apt to be a little over-exacting, and to drive her friends rather hard. Also she did not relish independence or opposition. "I like being under obedience to you," wrote one of her nursing friends, always very dear to her. Not indeed that Miss Nightingale had any weakness for gush—no one had less; but if a friend was other-wise admirable to her—by good sense and zeal, and so forth, the fact of the "obedience" was not other than an additional recommendation. She was inclined to resent any diversion on the part of her friends to other interests as desertion.

All this will, I think, sometimes be felt to be true by those who read the present Memoir. Yet it is only part of the truth; and because the final truth resides in the whole it is in a sense not true at all. The greatness of Miss Nightingale's character, and the secret of her life's work, consist in the union of qualities not often found in the same man or woman. She was not a sentimentalist; yet she was possessed by an infinite compassion. Pity for the sick and sorrowful,—a passionate desire to serve them,—devotion to her "children," the common soldiers—sym-pathy with the voiceless peasants of India: these were ruling motives of her life. She scorned those who were "only enthusiasts"; but there was no height of devotion to which a considered enthusiasm would not lead her. She had in equal measure cleverness and charm. She had a pungent wit, but also a loving heart. The sharpness often prominent in her letters was not always the expression of her real mind or manner. She shunned "the broad way and the green"; but Colonel Lefroy applied to her no less the later words: "they that overween, No anger find in thee, but pity and truth." She combined in a rare degree strength and tenderness. Masterful in action, she was humble, even to the verge of morbid abasement, in thought. She was at once Positive and Mystic. All this also will, as I hope, be found proven in the Memoir.

A curious, and a larger, question is raised by some of the apparent contradictions in Miss Nightingale's aim, thoughts, and character. She was intensely spiritual; she sought continually for the Kingdom of Heaven, and she conceived of it as a kingdom of the soul. Yet her aim may seem material; what she sought was a kingdom of more airy hos-pitals, more scientific nursing, brighter barracks, cleaner homes, better laid drains. It was after all a searching question which the Aga Khan put to her, as he listened to the tale of sanitary improvement during the fifty years of her active life. "But are your people better?" Are there more of them, we may conceive him as saying, who have attained to the kingdom of heaven in their souls? And unless you can show me that such has been the case, why have you, with your great influence and powers, devoted your life to this service of tables?

What reply she made to the Prince I do not know. The answer in her mind may be gathered from the course of her life, the nature of her speculations, and the bent of her character. At recurrent intervals she had formed thoughts for the main purposes of her life other than those which in fact she fulfilled. We have heard of her desire "to find a new religion for the artizans," and there are letters to Mr. Jowett in which she speaks of this desire—of the hope to establish on some sure foundation an organized creed and church—as the longing of her life. She had to abandon it, but never, in the most prosaic or material of her undertakings did she forget her spiritual ideals. She held, as her ideal of nursing shows, that "it takes a soul to raise a body even to a cleaner sty." She held also that the cleaner sty, though it might be the first thing needful, was not the end, but a means. "We must beware," she wrote, "both of thinking that we can maintain the 'Kingdom of Heaven within' under all circumstances,—because there are circumstances under which the human being cannot be good,—and also of thinking that the Kingdom of Heaven *without* will produce the Kingdom of Heaven within."

Miss Nightingale's own peculiar genius was for administration and order; and she had to employ her genius within the fields of opportunity which her sex and her circumstances offered. She was fond of quoting a passage which she found in one of Sir Samuel Baker's books of travel. "I, being unfortunately dependent on their movements, am more like a donkey than an explorer—that is, saddled and ridden away at a moment's notice." "I never did anything," she once said to a young friend, "except when I was asked." It will be agreed by all who have read this Memoir that Miss Nightingale interpreted her mandates in a spacious sense admitting of much initiative. Yet it is true in large measure that her work was the creation of circumstances, and was, in some fields, dependent on what she and Mr. Jowett used to call "temples of friendship" with political administrators.

Miss Nightingale's scope of action was thus limited; but the limits did not prevent the application of her fundamental ideas. "Perhaps," she wrote in one of her meditations (1868), "it is what I have seen of the misery and worthlessness of human life (few have seen more), together with the extraordinary power which God has put into the hands of quite ordinary people (if they would but use it) for raising mankind out of this misery and worthlessness, which has given me this intense and ever present feeling of an Eternal Life leading to perfection for each and for every one of us, by God's laws." Miss Nightingale did not suppose that human perfectibility, that the final union of man with God, was to be attained only by better sanitation. But she saw that this was the field open to her, and that it admitted of tilling by methods, which if applied to all departments of life would, as she conceived, lead to the one far-off Divine event. "Christianity," she wrote, "is to see God in

everything, to find Him out in everything, in the order or laws as of
His moral or spiritual, so of His political or social, and so of His physical worlds . . . To Christ God was everything—to us He seems nothing,
almost if not quite nothing, or if He is anything, He is only the God of
Sundays, and only the God of Sundays as far as going to what we call
our prayers, not the God of our week-days, our business, and our
play, our politics and our science, our home life and our social life;
our House of Commons, our Government, our post-office and correspondence—such an enormous item in these days—our Foreign Office,
and our Indian Office . . . The Kingdom of Heaven is within, but we
must also make it so without. There is no public opinion yet, it has to
be created, as to not committing blunders for want of knowledge;
good intentions are supposed enough; yet blunders—organized blunders—do more mischief than crimes . . . To study how to do good work,
as a matter of life or death; to 'agonise' so as to obtain practical wisdom to do it, there is little or no public opinion enforcing this—con-
demning the want of it. Until you can create such a public opinion
little good will be done, except by accident or by accidental individuals. But when we have such a public opinion, we shall not be far
from having a Kingdom of Heaven externally, even here." "I never
despair," she had written some years before, "that, in God's good
time, every one of us will reap the common benefit of obeying all the
laws which He has given us for our well-being." And towards that end,
it was the duty of each and all, according to their several opportunities,
to "work, work, work."

Having found her appointed corner in the vineyard, Miss Nightingale devoted her life to it; in equal measure, with careful adjustment
of means to ends, and with intense devotion. "To make an art of *Life!*"
she wrote to Madame Mohl (May 20, 1868). "That is the finest art of
all the Fine Arts. And few there be that find it. It was the 'one thing
wanting' to dear ——. She had the finest moral nature I ever knew.
Yet she never did any good to herself or to any one else. Because she
never could make Life an Art. I used sometimes to say to her:—*Do
you mean to go on in that way for twenty years?*—packing everybody's
carpet-bag. She always said she didn't. But she always did. And if she
did not go on for twenty years, it was only because Death came. I am
obliged (by my ill-health) to make Life an Art—to be always thinking
of it. Because otherwise I should do *nothing*. (I have so little life and
strength.)" Miss Nightingale had come back from the Crimea full of
honour. But she returned also seriously injured in health. How naturally
might a woman of less resolute character have rested on her laurels, and

sunk into a life of gracious repose or valetudinarian indolence! She chose, however, the better and the rougher path. She framed a regimen which shut her off from many of the common enjoyments of life, which to some degree impaired the flow of her domestic affections, but which enabled her, through nearly fifty years of recurrent weakness, to follow her highest ideals and to devote herself to work of public beneficence.

The circumstances of her life as they were ordered for her, the manner of her life as she framed it to meet them, led to some other traits of character which, again, present at first sight a curious contrariety. "She is extremely modest," said the Prince Consort and Queen Victoria when they met her, and she made the same impression on all who came in contact with her whether in the region of public affairs or in that of nursing. She had a consistent and a perfectly sincere shrinking from every form of popular glare and glory. There are passages, however, in letters to her intimate friends which leave, on a first reading, a somewhat different impression. She craved for a full and understanding sympathy with her mission and her work. She was fully conscious, it would seem, of her great powers; she did not always care, in private letters, to hide or to under-rate the extent of her influence upon men and affairs. She objected, in one letter to a friend, that Kinglake's chapter was intolerable because it posed her as "a Tragedy Queen"; but there are other letters in which she dramatizes herself somewhat; there is self-pity in them, and there is other self-consciousness. All this, which on a superficial glance may seem to present some difficult inconsistency, admits, I think, of easy explanation when the conditions of her life are remembered. She was intensely conscious of a special destiny, and the tenacity with which in the face of many obstacles she clung to her sense of a vocation enabled her to fulfil it. The sphere of women's work and opportunities has been so much widened in the present day, that readers of a generation later than Florence Nightingale's may require, perhaps, to make some effort of sympathetic imagination in order to realize how much of a pioneer she was. In her earlier years it was a daring novelty for a young woman to put her hand to any solid work in political administration or other organizing business. She knew all this by hard experience, and it emphasized her sense of special destiny. The manner of her life threw her at the same time, at each stage, though in different ways, in upon herself. During the thwarted years of her youth, she found little outlet except, as she said in "dreaming"; in dreaming, that is, of the things she might do, in imagining herself in this position of influence or in that. When the opportunity came to her of doing great things, not dreaming them, her youth and early womanhood were already past. Miss Nightingale was thirty-four when she went out to the Crimean war. In the later years, the conditions in which she lived again encouraged, almost of necessity, a habit of introspection: a habit which was also confirmed by her mystical view of the duty of living an inner life of conscious self-realization. Returning from the East in a state of nervous exhaustion, she was absorbed in work which could not wait. She was haunted for many years by threats of early death. There were such things to be, such things to do. But she did them for the most part in loneliness and without any habitual companionship. Except during the five years of almost daily converse with Sidney Herbert, she enjoyed none of that influence, at once sobering and fortifying, which comes from the equal clash of mind with mind. The result was a strain of morbidness which found occasional expression in notes of excessive self-consciousness.

There was, however, a more constant note. The nobility of Miss Nightingale's character and the worth of her life as an example are to be found, not least in the fundamental humility of temper and sanity of self-judgment which caused her to aim with consistent purpose, not only at great deeds, but at the doing of them from the highest motives. She never felt that she had done anything which might not have been done better; and, though she must have been conscious that she had done great things, she was forever examining her motives and finding them fall short of her highest ideals. There is a story told of a famous artist, that a friend entering his studio found him in tears. "I have produced a work," he said, "with which I am satisfied, and I shall never produce another." The premonition was true. No later masterpiece was produced. The inspiration of the ideal was gone. That inspiration never forsook Miss Nightingale in her pursuit of the art of life.

In life, as in other arts, what is spontaneous, and perhaps even what is unregenerate, have often more of charm than what is acquired or learnt by discipline. And in the case of Miss Nightingale, her elemental vigour of mind and force of will, will perhaps to some readers seem more admirable than the philosophy which she applied to her conduct or the acquired graces with which she sought to chasten her character. But however this may be, her constant striving after something which she deemed better, and the unceasing conflict which she waged, now with opposition of outward circumstance and now with undisciplined impulses from within, add savour and poignancy to her life.

No man knew her so well for so many years as Mr. Jowett, and the thought of her life never ceased to excite his admiration. "Most persons are engaged," he wrote at Christmas-time 1886, "in feasting and holiday-making amid their friends and relatives. You are alone in your room devising plans for the good of the natives of India or of the English soldiers as you have been for the last thirty years, and always deploring your failures as you have been doing for the last thirty years, though you have had a far greater and more real success in life than any other lady of your time." And again: "There are those who respect and love you, not for the halo of glory which surrounded your name in the Crimea, but for the patient toil which you have endured since on behalf of every one who is suffering or wretched." To us who are able to enter even more fully than Mr. Jowett into the inner life of Miss Nightingale, the respect and admiration may well be yet more enhanced, as we picture the conditions in which the patient toil was done, and remember the struggles of a beautifully sensitive soul in ascending the path towards perfection.

Such is the picture of Miss Nightingale which this Book has endeavoured to draw. As I wrote it I often thought with Mr. Jowett, that the life of the secluded worker in the solitary bedroom in South Street was more impressive even than the better known episodes of Santa Filomena in the fever-haunted wards of Scutari, or of the Lady-in-Chief giving her orders as she trudged through the snow from hut to hut on the heights of Balaclava. But it is Miss Nightingale herself who, unconsciously, has said the last words on her Life and Character. In praising one of her fellow-workers, and, next, in giving counsel to some fellow-seekers after good, she used phrases which may well be applied to herself:—

"One whose life makes a great difference for all: *all* are better off than if he had not lived; and this betterness is for always, it does not die with him—that is the true estimate of a great LIFE."

"Live your life while you have it. Life is a splendid gift. There is nothing small in it. For the greatest things grow by God's law out of the smallest. But to live your life, you must discipline it. You must not fritter it away in 'fair purpose, erring act, inconstant will'; but must make your thought, your words, your acts all work to the same end, and that end not self but God. This is what we call CHARACTER."

In the previous selection, Sir Edward T. Cook has provided
the most complete and most accepted portrait of Florence
Nightingale. Lytton Strachey notwithstanding, the interpretation has survived through the years with only Mrs.
Cecil Woodham-Smith making any significant additions.
Donald Allen, in the article reprinted here, contends,
however, that none of these authors or any others have
adequately explained her success. He therefore attempts
to supplement all previous work by applying the concepts
of psychoanalytic psychology to the many facets of
Florence Nightingale's character and life. Allen, a university
professor of History, seeks the causes for her behavior
through an examination of the basic conflicts of her personality and, in the process, offers explanations for certain
events or results that highlighted her life.

DONALD R. ALLEN

"Florence Nightingale: Toward a Psychohistorical Interpretation"

Florence Nightingale's life and career pose one demanding question
above all else: How did a woman in mid- and late Victorian England
achieve such formidable power and influence in so many areas of public
administration? History is in large part the story of change, and the
changes effected in this "age of reform" in public and private sanitation, in nursing, in the care and provisioning of the military, in the construction of hospitals, in the mighty War Office, and in the administration
of India—to name only Florence Nightingale's major preoccupations—
were often due directly to her efforts. Her public life, and a good part
of her private life, have long been open to the public gaze; indeed, it
would be difficult to find another woman in modern times about whom
more has been written. Yet, it seems that Florence Nightingale's success
has never been adequately explained.

The present investigation makes no pretense of supplanting the
major studies of Florence Nightingale's life and career. Rather, it is an
attempt to supplement these works by applying to them some of the

concepts of psychoanalytic psychology. In this way it serves as a response to White's complaint that in an age when rationality, insight, and creative social invention are in urgent demand, little has been provided in the way of systematic case records of great fortitude, rare heroism, or special success in grasping and solving important social issues. His complaint has special validity concerning women. The main theme of this study is that Florence Nightingale achieved greatness through her efforts to control the basic conflicts of her personality which affected her finding her niche in society. Her success in accomplishing this objective was only reached at high cost in each of the stages of her life, but the result was a unique and personally satisfying contribution of no small measure.

An understanding of Florence Nightingale's personality first requires a brief outline of her family constellation, of the attitude toward women in early and mid-Victorian society, and of the prevailing attitudes toward nursing as a profession, especially for women of high station. She was born on 12 May 1820, the younger daughter of William E. and Frances Smith Nightingale. The birth of the Nightingales' only children, two daughters, came during a long sojourn in Italy, and both were named after their birthplaces. The elder, born in Naples in 1819, was named Frances Parthenope, Frances after her mother and Parthenope after the old Greek settlement on the site of Naples.

Both families in the Nightingale marriage belonged to the moneyed and propertied Whig gentry. William Nightingale came from the old Derbyshire family of Shore of Tapton and changed his name in 1815 to Nightingale on succeeding to the property of his mother's uncle, Peter Nightingale of Lea. He was educated at Edinburgh University and Trinity College, Cambridge, and was fond of travel, having made the grand tour of the Continent shortly after the Napoleonic wars. As an active supporter of parliamentary reform, he was a follower of Bentham and, later, Lord Palmerston, who was a neighbor in the country. At his wife's urging he stood for a seat in the House of Commons in 1835, and lost. His idealism bruised, he then refused to take any further active role in politics, indulging instead his preference for country life, local affairs, long solitary rides in the New Forest, speculation along religious and philosophical lines, and the education of his daughters.

The marriage was not a particularly happy one, although William Nightingale had been deeply in love with his new wife, six years his senior and the elder sister of one of his school friends. To his daughters he appeared as a rather warm and sympathetic figure, though not as a

particularly strong one. Later an alliance system developed which found
William Nightingale siding with Florence, his prize pupil, against her
mother and Parthe, especially over the question of Florence's independence. Yet in Florence's eyes, he was only mildly supportive in this
role as in others: *"Effleurez, n'appuyez pas* has been not the rule but
the habit of his life," she later wrote. It would appear, however, that
the lightness of the father's touch was made up for by the heaviness
of the mother's.

Frances (Fanny) Smith had married William Nightingale only a
year after falling in love with a younger son of the Early of Caithness, a
match rejected by her father because of the suitor's lack of an adequate
income or expectations. Although she did not marry until age 29, Fanny
was considered the beauty of a large, rich, and socially prominent
family. Her father, William Smith, sat in Parliament for forty-six years
as a champion of abolition, factory workers, dissenters, and Jews. His
ten children did not take up these interests but concentrated on their
social talents and activities. Fanny's ambition was to become a great
hostess, to mold her husband into one of the prosperous, cultivated,
and liberal-minded country gentlemen, like her father, who played an
important part in English public life. When this plan misfired in the
elections of 1835, having no sons, she transferred her social ambitions
to her daughters. In the family constellation Fanny became allied with
her elder daughter against her husband and Florence; the lines were
clearly discernible by the time of Florence's adolescence. Florence
Nightingale's greatest agony concerned her inability to accept her
mother's irreducible ideas of the kind of life which she should lead and
the unhappiness and vexation this inability caused her mother.

Parthe was the elder (by one year), the plainer, the less gifted, in
all, the less remarkable daughter. The relationship between the sisters
was marked by a strong sibling rivalry which played a role in blocking
full personality development for both of them. At age 48 Florence still
referred to Parthe as "always, as she always had been the spoilt child."
Florence early emerged as the leader and Parthe followed resentfully.
Parthe fluctuated between passionate attachment to Florence and extreme vexation with her, enough so that their parents thought it prudent
to send the two children to different branches of the family for holi-
days. While Florence responded well to her father's educating endeavors,
Parthe reacted with boredom and a growing sense of distance between
her father and herself. By age 16 she had joined with her mother in
strictly feminine interests in the drawing-room and the garden, and later
aided in her mother's decades-long efforts—with hysterics and illness—to

make Florence "stay at home" and give up her dreams of a career in nursing. Parthe relinquished her hold on her younger sister only after her own marriage at age 39. Up to this point the more attractive suitors, the better looks, the more brilliant conversations, and the fame had largely belonged to her sister. Florence and Parthe became fully reconciled and returned to their childhood intimacy only after their parents' death and when Parthe was almost hopelessly crippled by arthritis. She died in 1890 at age 71, some twenty years before the death of Florence.

The Nightingale family constellation was marked, therefore, by several disturbing features: an ambitious and domineering mother who soon became estranged from her difficult younger daughter, a relatively weak father, an enduring alliance system, and intense sibling rivalry. These features alone would be serious enough to affect Florence's psychosexual and psychosocial development; joined with Victorian attitudes toward women, they amounted to a formidable barrier to the achievement of the goal for which she felt herself fated.

Today the lot of the Victorian middle-class woman would seem essentially unhappy, if, as in the case of Florence Nightingale, she rebelled against the standards of the time. The woman's world was strictly confined to the interests of home and family, and the only truly acceptable roles were, progressively, those of dutiful daughter, obedient wife, and protective mother. A spinster might be accommodated as a kind of higher-level servant at the beck and call of a thousand family needs. In fact, many women in upper stations did not marry, but it was in few ways a desirable situation. The rigidly defined parameters for the "perfect lady" were most fully developed in the upper middle class, where her upbringing combined total sexual innocence, conspicuous consumption, and the worship of the family hearth. When she married, the perfect lady simply transferred her loyalties and values from her father's home to that of her husband.

That home life held no attraction for Florence Nightingale is perfectly clear from her writings; her indictment of life in a Victorian family, for all of the warmth and affection to be found there, is probably unsurpassed in its depth and feeling:

> O weary days—oh evenings that seem never to end—and for how many years have I watched that drawing-room clock and thought it never would reach ten! and for twenty, thirty years more to do this!
>
> 'Butchered to make a Roman Holiday.' Women don't consider themselves as human beings at all. There is absolutely no God, no country, no duty to them at all except family. . . . I have known a good deal of convents. And

of course everyone has talked of the petty grinding tyrannies supposed to be exercised there. But I know nothing like the petty grinding tyranny of a good English family. And the only alleviation is that the tyrannized submits with a heart full of affection.

For Florence Nightingale the alternative to oppressive home life was nursing; yet that choice presented even further problems. Southwood Smith's remark in the 1840s that "the generality of nurses in hospitals are not such as the medical men can place much confidence in" was surely a discreet understatement for a deplorable situation. Nursing in the mid-Victorian period was associated with menial domestic work and in no way considered a profession suited to "respectable" women. It was ill-paid, no high standard of efficiency was expected, and formal training was virtually non-existent. Low morality and a wanton life-style were other characteristics associated with nursing. A doctor in the North wrote in answer to a circular concerning the use of nurses, "If I can but obtain a sober set, it is as much as I can hope for." Florence Nightingale herself, after many observations, stated that hospitals were "as school . . . for immorality and impropriety—inevitable where women of bad character are admitted as nurses, to become worse by their contact with male patients and young surgeons." In light of such evidence, and the fact that it was unthinkable for upper-class Victorian women to go "out to work," the hostile reaction of Florence Nightingale's family to her desire for a career in nursing is not surprising; nor is it surprising that the dutiful daughter took eight years of tremendous mental anguish to break her family bonds and realize her ambitions.

Five periods in Florence Nightingale's life call for special attention, for in each of these periods one can recognize a turning point, marked by an internal crisis, that led to a new stage in her development. Chronologically they are: her childhood development to about age 7; the "call from God" which she experienced at age 16; her decision, following a long moratorium at home, to renounce marriage and her family to pursue an independent course, a decision which resolved her long crisis of identity; her alliance with Sidney Herbert following her return from the Crimean War, which gave her access to power and defined her work style for her most productive and creative period; and, finally, the death of her parents and sister, which freed her from a lifelong conflict and permitted her to enter a long period at the end of her life when, her fury abated, she enjoyed the fruits of her labors and contributions.

Florence Nightingale's entire life carried the strain of conflict with her mother who ever opposed her finding her own identity. Florence, in turn, was torn between love for her mother, which she felt was never recognized, and desire for her own life. The attachment to her mother ended early. Florence was an unhappy child, not naughty, but strange, obstinate, and ready to attach herself passionately to any other female— to Miss Christie (her governess), to Aunt Mai (Mrs. Samuel Smith, her father's younger sister), to a beautiful older cousin. When they left, "the violence of her feelings made her physically ill." To her parents she seemed an unhappy child who was difficult to understand, a girl who had consciously rebelled against her life since age 6. Her mother was especially perplexed by the attitude of this "wild swan we have hatched," and her father wrote when she was twelve: "Ask Flo if she has lost her intellect. If not, why does she grumble at troubles which she cannot remedy by grumbling?"

In a significant, private autobiographical note later in life, Florence Nightingale recalled the pain and difficulty of her childhood years. Writing of the time when she was about six years old she revealed that she had an obsession that she was some kind of "monster," different from other people and frightened that they might find out her "secret." The prospect of seeing a new face was agony, and she refused to dine downstairs with the rest of the family because "I had a morbid terror of not using my knives and forks like other people when I should come out." There was also a great fear of meeting children, "because I was sure I should not please them." Not surprisingly, she often escaped into "dreaming," and for long hours at a time she transferred herself completely to a dream world where she saw herself in the role of a heroine, a habit that stayed with her through her early adult life.

The argument can be made that the sense of basic trust which Erikson posits as the fundamental prerequisite for mental vitality and which depends on the quality of the maternal relationship was somehow aborted in Florence Nightingale. Erikson points out that the guilt aroused by childhood moralism leads to consequences that often do not appear until much later "when conflicts over initiative may find expression in a self-restriction." This may keep an individual from living up to his inner capacities or "to the powers of his imagination and feeling (if not [resulting] in relative sexual impotence or frigidity)." In turn, the individual may overcompensate and show "tireless initiative," a "go-at-it-iveness at all cost." Florence's early unhappiness and childhood moralism were reflected in her adult life along the lines suggested by Erikson. Her family had to be held at bay lest they interfere with her work; her relationship with her closest friend, Mary Clarke Mohl, worked only because Mme. Mohl lived in Paris and they saw each other infrequently; a self-restricted sexuality was irrevocably determined by her final rejection of Richard Monckton Milnes' long devotion and proposal of marriage in 1849—she had already rejected other proposals—despite her assertion that she loved him and that he was acceptable in every way; and, as we shall see, she consistently experienced deep feelings of failure in spite of and even at the apex of her greatest achievements. In short, a discrepancy existed between her low self-esteem and high ego ideal. Her attempts to deal with this discrepancy took the direction of fantasy and, increasingly, action.

The development of Florence's sense of autonomy also seems to have been impaired, which may explain in part her heightened sense of shame as a child. There is some evidence that Florence's lifelong estrangement from her mother might have been involved with her sexual development. Certainly Fanny saw her younger daughter's later rebellion in sexual terms. When Florence announced in 1845 that she wished to be trained as a nurse, her mother reacted with a terror that quickly turned to rage as she accused Florence of having "an attachment of which she was ashamed," a secret love life with some "low vulgar surgeon." As Florence wrote to her cousin,

> ...I thought something like a Protestant Sisterhood, without vows, for women of educated feelings, might be established. But there have been difficulties about my very first step, which terrified Mama. I do not mean the physically revolting parts of a hospital, but things about the surgeons and nurses which you may guess.

A few years later when she rejected Milnes' proposal of marriage her mother accused her of "godless ingratitude, perversity, and conceit," extremely strong comments which revealed the depth of Fanny's feelings.

Another reason for the conflict between mother and daughter—and for Florence's feeling of rejection and acquisition of "masculine" characteristics—may lie in Fanny's wish for a son. A son was especially desired by the Nightingales because a good part of the fortune of William Nightingale would pass on his death to his younger sister and then to her son if William did not have a direct male heir. That Florence accepted a man's education from her father was perhaps partly a wish to satisfy her mother. In a happier moment she even wrote an imaginary speech to her mother in which she begged to be regarded as a son, a masculine self-image that persisted in her work relationships throughout life. "You must look at me as your vagabond son," she wrote, "Remember, I should have cost you a great deal more if I had been married or a son. You were willing enough to part with me to be married."

The estrangement from her mother led Florence to form strong attachments not only to surrogate mothers but also, quite naturally, to her father. At the same time, Parthe retained her own intimate tie with Fanny and began a lifelong relationship with Florence that alternated between Parthe's passionate over-attachment and long estrangement between the sisters. Florence suffered intensely from what she saw as a rejection brought on by her own willfulness: "I thought I would go up to the Eumenides Cave," she wrote poignantly in Greece in 1850, "and ask God there to explain to me what were these Eumenides which pursued me. I would not ask to be relieved of them—welcome, Eumenides—but to be delivered from doing further wrong. Orestes himself did not go on murdering." The strong mixture of narcissism and masochism engendered by family conflict and reflected here accounts in part for the aggressive nature of her work style later on.

The alliance between Florence and her father intensified as her education came under his supervision. As a liberal Unitarian and Whig, William Nightingale held advanced ideas on the education of women and felt that no tutor could provide his daughters with the kind of education that he thought was necessary in the new age of enlightened liberalism. In fact, however, it might be suggested that his educational endeavors with his daughters constituted in large part a working out of his desire for a son. They were, in effect, given a thoroughly "modern" and "masculine" education which included instruction in French, German, Italian, history, philosophy, and classical Greek and Latin. Florence responded well to the rigorous hours and taxing schedule; Parthe, although bright, rebelled and escaped to her mother. By the time Florence was sixteen the lines were drawn: Florence and her father in the library, Parthe and her mother in the drawing room.

The close relationship between father and younger daughter proved extremely advantageous to Florence when she made her decision to pursue a career in nursing. Although not pleased with her intention, he did not oppose it with the vehemence and force of Fanny and Parthe, and when in 1851 her first opportunity for employment presented itself in the form of the superintendency of the Institution for the Care of Sick Gentlewomen in Distressed Circumstances William Nightingale quickly and quietly provided Florence with an allowance of £500 a year which secured her personal independence. He also told her to write to him privately at his club in order to circumvent the Nightingale family practice of passing around all letters. When Florence later took up her philosophical and religious speculations in a serious way, William again became her confidant and "sat at her feet and sympathized in her searches after truth." Yet, this was not enough for Florence, who did not regard her father as sufficiently supportive; but then, nobody was. "My father," she wrote just before gaining her independence, "is a man who has never known what struggle is. Good impulses from his childhood up, and always remaining perfectly in a natural state, acting always from impulse—and never having by circumstances been forced to look into a thing, to carry it out."

This picture of Florence Nightingale's psychosexual and psychosocial development in her childhood years corresponds rather closely to certain characteristics and personality traits described by Deutsch in her treatment of feminine masochism and the "masculinity complex" in the "active woman." Deutsch points out that although it is normal for the girl to turn away from the mother and childhood dependencies in favor of active adjustment to reality as represented by the father, this adjustment, or reaction formation, entails negative feelings of hostility toward the mother (to overcome fear of losing her), which in favorable cases ends with a positive, tender, and forgiving relation with the mother. Such a relation is one of the most important prerequisites for psychological harmony in later femininity. In certain cases, however, a split may occur at a very early age. The girl's active sublimating tendencies become attached to the father, while her sexual fantasies "assume an extraordinarily passive and masochistic character," which characterizes her later sexual behavior; this type of woman either remains erotically isolated, avoiding all dangers—like Florence Nightingale—or falls victim to brutal men. In this situation "the feminine erotic component remains on the level of infantile masochism," the woman's attitude toward life may be very active and masculine, and "[she] may display particular resistance and aggressiveness in the struggle for life." Feminine masochism may also be reflected in the willingness to serve a cause or a human being with love and abnegation—the kind of activity Florence undertook at an early age with sick relatives and with her mother among the poor and sick villagers of the neighborhood. Later it assumed massive proportions in her love for the British soldier, her disdain for her personal health and safety in the Crimea, her lifelong dedication to her cause, and her scorn for public acclaim. Here a compromise is effected between masochism and narcissism, between self-injury and self-love, "just like the erotic type of woman in her more normal manner."

That a strong masochistic strain existed in Florence Nightingale, which helped her to choose and pursue a career in nursing, seems clear. The failure to resolve her conflict with her mother; the "inhibiting" education by her father along the lines then associated with boys; the strong and sometimes secret alliance with her father which may have prevented her from successfully completing her psychosexual development; her unhappiness as a child with escapes to a dream world and a morbid fear of being "found out"; the failure to achieve true personal erotic intimacy—all converged in a renewed aspiration, laden with masochistic elements, to go forward aggressively. This aspiration was funneled into an all-consuming passion to enter nursing and by so doing to create a unique identity and life style that would calm the conflicts within her.

Florence Nightingale's choice of nursing as a career brings us to the second turning point in her psychosocial and psychosexual development: a religious crisis in which she experienced a "call from God" directing her to a special destiny. This crisis began her long search for a career, which was partly resolved in her decision to pursue nursing, and culminated, in her early 30s, in an "identity crisis" whereupon she rejected marriage, won independence from her family, and began her productive life. This period served as a kind of moratorium when destructive and constuctive forces battled within her and regressive and progressive alternatives presented themselves. Two questions call for special attention in this stage: What was the nature of her call and how did her religious ideas fit with her overall development? And why did this religious experience direct her toward nursing?

In a private note to herself written in 1867, Florence Nightingale revealed that just before she turned seventeen, she underwent a religious experience akin to that of Joan of Arc: "on February 7th, 1837, God spoke to me and called me to His service." This was not an inward revelation but an "objective" voice, outside of herself, speaking to her in human words. She laters stated that her "voices" had spoken to her on four occasions: On the date of her call at Embley; once in 1853 before going to her first position at the hospital for poor gentlewomen in Harley Street; once before her departure for the Crimea in 1854; and once after the death of Sidney Herbert, her closest collaborator, in 1861. All of these experiences with "voices" occurred after periods of extremely intense emotional and psychological stress marked by personal disappointment, strong feelings of self-doubt, deep depression, and a sense of failure. In turn, all were followed by a strong desire to accomplish something, a devotion to work, and some kind of fulfillment.

Florence Nightingale's religious ideas and writings deserve a chapter in their own right; not only are the private and published materials quite extensive, but they are also revealing in the sense of being the product of an intensely introspective and spiritual figure with a high degree of intelligence and unflagging energy. Although there is no place here for any detailed treatment of her religious ideas, several elements should be noted because they relate to an understanding of her psychological makeup. First, there was a distinct "mystical" element as seen in her proclivity for introspection, in her conversion at age 16, and in her three subsequent experiences with "voices." Second, there was an overwhelming emotional and psychological need, sanctioned by and seen in terms of religious impulse, to devote her life to the care of the sick, which by age 24 had culminated in a decision to follow a nursing career at all cost. Third, in all of her religious thinking and writing there is little particular interest in doctrine or dogma, but rather a nearly exclusive concentration on "works" as the only criteria for the validity and purpose of religion, i.e., the testing of religious doctrine by practical results. As she once remarked to Richard Monckton Milnes, "It will never do unless we have a Church of which the terms of membership shall be works, not doctrines." Fourth, she suffered from a profound sense of guilt, expressed in terms of sin, which plagued her for most of her life. "Bless me, too, as poor Esau said," she wrote to Harriet Nicholson on Christmas Eve 1845. "I have *so* felt with him and cried with an exceeding bitter cry 'Bless me, even me also, Oh my father,' but He never has yet and I have not deserved that He should." One final aspect of her religious thought concerns her conception of the nature of God. She was not drawn to the figure of Jesus or the doctrines of salvation, redemption, and the incarnation of Christ. Rather she looked to God the Father, who wished his children to follow His absolute moral laws and do His work for the relief of misery. This primary alliance with God alone provided her with the sense of strength to unlock the chains which bound her, and it became the source of her tremendous tenacity and willpower.

The religious impulses moving Florence during these years formed but a part, albeit an important one, of the decisive stage in her life when she came to grips with her identity and definitively mapped her future course in life. Her crisis of identity opened with her "call" at age 16 and closed—in the sense of her having defined her adult psychosocial and psychosexual style and being able to go on to her most creative and productive period—between her thirtieth and thirty-second years. By its end, she had come to believe totally in the uniqueness of her particular role in life; she had settled upon nursing as her profession; she had renounced marriage as a way of life acceptable to her (or to her nurses); and she had resolved to break the restraints imposed on her by her parents and sister.

In other ways, of course, her identity crisis was not "closed" at all, for problems which seemed momentarily solved reappeared later in new or familiar guises or had far-reaching results. Florence Nightingale failed, for example, to achieve true intimacy—either sexually, or, in Erikson's words, as "a true and mutual psychosocial intimacy with another person, be it in a friendship, in erotic encounters, or in joint inspiration." There were, indeed, close personal relationships and collaborations, such as those with Selina Bracebridge, who helped pry Florence loose from her mother and later accompanied her to the Crimea; with her closest partner in reform after the Crimean experience, Secretary of State for War Sidney Herbert; and with Benjamin Jowett, the Oxford classicist who became a great source of inspiration and consolation to her. But just as in childhood with her surrogate mothers, she could brook no hint in these intense relationships of "betrayal" or abandonment.

Two examples will suffice to show the extent of her insecurity. With her gift to command loyalty and devotion she literally worked her closest collaborator, Sidney Herbert, to death, while at the same time castigating the dying man ummercifully. When he was forced to resign from the War Office in 1861 because of a breakdown in health, Florence would have none of it. "No man in my day has thrown away so noble a game with all the winning cards in his hands," she wrote, although two months later Herbert was dead. Another example occurred in 1860 with her oldest and dearest friend, "Aunt Mai," who, after having left her own family for four years (1857-1860) to live with and care for Florence, decided she must go home; her husband had become virtually a stranger and her second daughter was to be married. The bitterness that her departure provoked in Florence was intense and unreasonable. When she realized that Aunt Mai was leaving, Florence refused to speak to or see her, nor would she forgive her for twenty years, during which time they never met and the correspondence between them ceased. There can be little doubt that the total blocking of her natural sex drives, finalized by her refusal of Monckton Milnes' marriage proposal but reaching back to her childhood experiences, could only prevent her from arriving at that true interpersonal intimacy in adult life described by Erikson as crucial to a "vital" personality.

The danger of the identity crisis stage is that of identity confusion or role confusion, which most often centers on the inability to choose an occupational identity:

> A state of acute identity confusion usually becomes manifest at a time when the young individual finds himself exposed to a combination of experiences which demand his simultaneous commitment to physical intimacy (not by any means always overtly sexual), to decisive occupational choice, to energetic competition, and to psychosocial self-definition. Whether or not the ensuing tension will lead to paralysis now depends primarily on the regressive pull exerted by a latent illness . . . The social functioning of the state of paralysis which ensues is that of maintaining a state of minimal choice and commitment.

Florence Nightingale experienced an extended moratorium marked by deep depressive states. Her "call" came in 1837, but it did not say what to do. Eight years passed until she decided what her vocation was, and the interval between the decision in 1844 to devote her life to nursing and her gaining freedom to pursue it lasted another eight years. The exciting trip to the continent and the enduring friendship with Mary Clarke Mohl, the tempting and brilliant series of balls and parties back in England, the flattering attentions of attractive suitors, all quickly paled in the face of her sense of frustration, confusion, and the lack of power to affect her own destiny. The personal notes poured out her increasing bitterness and despair in tens of thousands of words: "This morning I felt as if my soul would pass away in tears, in utter loneliness in a bitter passion of tears and agony of solitude." "I cannot live— forgive me, oh Lord, and let me die, this day let me die." These statements date from 1845, just after the realization that her future life lay in nursing and while she was still playing the role of the faithful "daughter at home." They mark the profoundest depth of her depression and emanate from her parents' refusal to permit her to go to a hospital for training. Having plumbed these depths, however, she began the long upward struggle. It was often marked by disappointment and frustration, but by 1853 she found the strength to reintegrate the strands of her identity, make the decisions to break with family and suitor, and funnel her energies into productive and satisfying work.

The ties that bound Florence Nightingale during these years could have been broken only at immense emotional cost. Her failure to make the break points up the kind of severe identity confusion that Erikson describes, the characteristics of which in Florence Nightingale included an acute self-consciousness, the strain of tentative engagement with others, a severe upset in the sense of workmanship, and scornful hostility toward the roles offered by her family and society as proper and desirable. Her difficulty in stabilizing her ego identity, largely due to the conflict connected with the freeing of personal relationships, constituted a severe blockage in her development—in some ways, permanent—and is best revealed in her attitude toward her mother and sister.

As the "daughter at home" or in the presence of Fanny and Parthe, Florence was always a child, until she finally succeeded in banishing them from her presence in London in 1858 by means of a manipulated "illness." Only then was she free to pursue her interests unimpeded by their well-meaning but stifling and inconsiderate over-protectiveness. The blockage was not entirely removed until Fanny, and later Parthe, old and in ill health, became entirely dependent on Florence, at which point she assumed supervision of their households and their care. Moreover, although the choice at age 24 of a career in nursing and its subsequent realization may have contributed to the stabilization of Florence's ego identity to the point of permitting her to break her family bonds, it was not sufficient to give her complete mental and emotional peace. Nursing as a profession, with its masochistic overtones, probably served as an important sponge to absorb her fury, but it did not totally obliterate her hatred nor completely resolve her conflict. That state of peace required the unraveling—by their dependence and death—of the ties which bound her to her mother and sister. Before dealing with the later stages of her life, however, it is necessary to survey the workings of her professional life, which carried in it the strains of her previous personal development.

When she returned from the Crimean War in 1856 Florence Nightingale was obsessed by a sense of failure. In the eyes of the world hers was the greatest of triumphs for a woman in modern times, but she saw none of it. The obstructions placed in her path by an offended military officialdom—the enduring of petty recriminations, false accusations, and impossible conditions—and the attacks of cholera, dysentery, and rheumatism, united to weaken her both physically and emotionally. What especially haunted her was the realization that the same system that had slaughtered soldiers by the thousands in the Crimea—the health administration of the British Army—continued to do so around the world. She also realized, in an almost desperate way, that to effect reform of the system meant immediate action. Yet she was so ill, "it seemed madness to contemplate work. She found difficulty in breathing, suffered from palpitations, and was overcome by nausea at the sight of food." She fully expected to die shortly, a belief that remained constant for more than twenty years. Therefore her need was to find somebody to carry on the work: a man who would be acceptable to the official world, who would carry weight in high circles, yet who would be ready to submit to and be taught by her.

Florence Nightingale found her ideal collaborator in Sidney except that the mantle was never passed on because she out-lived him by more than fifty years. As Secretary of State at War during the Crimean War, Herbert was responsible for the provisioning and equipping of the British forces and had chosen Florence for the Scutari mission. He was an acquaintance of several years, came from the same social background, and was as well connected as anybody in public life. Moreover, he was a partisan of reform. Sidney Herbert formed part of that small band of men whose lives and careers became enmeshed with Florence Nightingale's cause, and whose devotion was illustrated by their total subjection to their acknowledged leader. The work style of Florence Nightingale is therefore elucidated by two factors: her illness, and her power to attract talented and powerful collaborators totally committed to her personally and to her cause.

In spite of her illness, an invitation from Queen Victoria to meet privately impelled Florence Nightingale to a burst of activity. She met with Lord Panmure, the Secretary for War, who agreed to set up a Royal Commission. The weakness and nausea continued, but Florence was able to work night and day preparing material for her interviews as *éminence grise* of the Commission, while in her few free hours she visited and inspected barracks, hospitals, and other institutions. The inner circle for preparation of the Royal Commission to Enquire into the Sanitary Condition of the Army consisted of Florence Nightingale (whom the others called the Commander-in-Chief), Sidney Herbert, and Dr. John Sutherland. She was able to make these men, as well as their wives, her willing slaves through a combination of incredible charm, totally unreasonable demands, and her health. When Dr. Sutherland was late with a report one evening, for example, he consented at her insistence to stay and complete it. After reading it she was not satisfied and sent a message to his home in Highgate demanding his immediate return for rewriting. When he lost his temper and refused, she collapsed into an "agitated half-fainting state." The call went out again to Highgate, since Dr. Sutherland was also her physician, and he came immediately expressing "great sorrow and penitence." Moreover, while constantly stressing her own maladies, she had contempt for the illnesses of those working closely with her. She pressed hard on Dr. Sutherland and even harder on the dying Sidney Herbert. To her their complaints were "fancies."

In 1857 her health gave way from overwork and she collapsed. She refused to go home to Embley or to be nursed—dependency was no longer acceptable—but instead insisted on taking a cure at Malvern, alone except for one footman. She was generally thought to be dying: Harriet Martineau even brought up to date her obituary notice for the *Daily Mail*. This collapse in August 1857 marked the beginning of Florence Nightingale's retirement into invalidism; she now began to use her illness as protection against her family and any unwanted attention. During that year her mother and sister had moved into the Burlington Hotel, where Florence had rooms, and they completely disrupted her life. When Parthe proposed coming to London in the winter as well, and Aunt Mai's letters could not prevent it, Florence had an "attack" consisting of "excessive hurried breathing with pain in the head and the heart"; this kept Parthe away. Another attempt in 1858 met with the same response. Aunt Mai successfully argued that while Florence's life "hung by a thread" it was too much for the family to expect to see her; they must stay away. By the summer of 1858 Parthe was engaged and abandoned her siege, as did Fanny. Florence was now left alone, her privacy guarded by Aunt Mai and Arthur Hugh Clough, Aunt Mai's son-in-law. Although Florence only ventured from her rooms twice in 1858, she continued to receive eminent visitors, especially if they could be of use, such as the Queen of Holland, the Crown Prince of Prussia, and the Duke of Cambridge.

Sidney Herbert's health gave way in 1858 but Florence refused to take notice. As she saw it, her function was to drive him on, and she was able to enlist Mrs. Herbert in the endeavor as well. Despite his declining health, Herbert accepted an appointment as Minister for War in 1859 in Palmerston's government, and he and Florence Nightingale together undertook to reform the War Office, an immensely laborious job. She approached this task almost with despair, dwelling on her self-sacrifice, her suffering, and the inadequacies of her collaborators. Never was there any expression of concern for Herbert's suffering, or even the realization that it could be serious. It is curious and even ironic that a woman whose name is most closely connected with the alleviation of human suffering, and who seemingly required great personal suffering in order to work at peak efficiency, had so little understanding of the pain and misery of those close to her.

After a long and arduous battle with kidney disease, Sidney Herbert died in 1861. According to his wife, his last words were "Poor

Florence, poor Florence, our joint work unfinished." When she received the news, grief, anger, frustration, and guilt all combined in Florence to cause another collapse which lasted four weeks. Yet her reaction had as its primary focus not the personal loss of a dear and devoted friend whom she had seen almost daily for years, but what that loss entailed for her work. "My work, the object of my life, the means to do it, all in one depart with him." Even God was in part to blame: It would have been "but to set aside a few trifling physical laws to save him." She never blamed herself for the debilitating effect of her anger on him; nor did she admit that she had worked him—and others—to death. Yet, a remarkable transformation took place in her. With the death of Herbert their positions became reversed: She, who had always been the teacher, the leader, now became the faithful disciple, the servant who only loved him; he, the student, the instrument, now became her "Master," the object of love and praise. "I loved and served him as no one else," she wrote to Sir John McNeill, one of their collaborators.

Her work, however, was far from over. She returned to activity, although now her isolation was practically complete. She soon undertook her greatest task, the peak of her working life—the Royal Commission on the Health of the Army in India. The tons of materials that she gathered and analyzed for the project filled two vans when she moved. She achieved great success, though any hint of failure or defeat brought back the symptoms of her illness. By 1865 she would see nobody not directly connected with her work, not even her oldest and dearest friend, Mary Clarke Mohl, or the Queen of Holland. Only her spiritual advisor, the Oxford classicist Benjamin Jowett, was allowed to call, and he was seldom in London.

From the experiences related above, a close connection between Florence Nightingale's work style and her illness can be inferred. The latter was most likely psychoneurotic, a defense mechanism tied both to her vexed relations with her family and to her consuming struggle for professional success. Her illness was at once a means of warding off the emotional conflict engendered by the interference of her mother and sister, and at the same time a mechanism which allowed her to become the object of their solicitous attention, and thus to overcome her childhood feeling of rejection. A consuming struggle for success, as White has pointed out, sometimes carried "the latent meaning of a vital personal vindication, a denial of inferiorities that had produced rage and panic in childhood." That this element had a role in Florence Nightingale's career can be seen both in her extreme vulnerability to even the smallest hint that her success was incomplete and in her relentless drive to make her triumph perfect. The achievement of her aspirations brought only temporary relief from her physical and emotional pain. No matter how great her success, whenever it was threatened or in any way diluted she reverted to despair, and the symptoms of her illness became aggravated. A willingness to accept less than complete victory in a project, and to gain relative satisfaction, came to her only late in life after her family conflict was resolved and her old collaborators were all dead.

In her sixties a significant change came over Florence Nightingale as the final definition of her personality took form, and it lasted until her death at the age of ninety. Her parents were now both dead, and her lifelong depressions seemed to pass. She became completely reconciled with Parthe, who was ill and required looking after, and the pervading benevolence that had often marked her young womanhood returned. Failure weighed less heavily and the self-reproaches ceased. "I cannot remember the time," she wrote to her friend Clarkey (Mary Clarke Mohl) in 1881,

> when I have not longed for death. After Sidney Herbert's death and [Arthur Hugh] Clough's death in 1861, 20 years ago, for years and years I used to watch for death as no sick man ever watched for the morning. It is strange that now bereft of all, I crave for it less. I want to do a little work, a little better, before I die.

Although opportunities presented themselves in both the War Office and the government of India, and she continued to work, it was no longer in a rage. When the tide turned against her now, as it did within a few years, it bothered her little. As she accepted old age, tolerance replaced the lifelong drive for perfection. Although her mind remained keen and her energy remarkable, she was no longer driven, and the last twenty years of her life were marked by warm relations with young relatives and student nurses of the Nightingale Training School, and by serenity and contentment. The last thirty years of her life were thus relatively happy. She was finally freed from the conflicts of her past, she enjoyed good health, and she was able to look back on her accomplishments with a sense of quiet pleasure and satisfaction.

Although Florence Nightingale was no ordinary person, as her achievements attest, the problems which she encountered were, for the most part, the same faced by an Victorian woman of her station who wished to create an independent and productive life outside of the prescribed progression of family, marriage, children, and discreet private charity: hostility, lack of understanding, and the realization of being out of tune with one's times. Moreover, the choice of nursing as the means to administrative power involved its own peculiar difficulties.

To understand Florence Nightingale's choice of nursing as a career and her development in accumulating and exercising power requires a recognition of the importance of conflict in her personality. The key to her conflict is her lifelong struggle with shame, or as she termed it, her "pride," a struggle which was probably the primary force for her drive toward accomplishment. When thirty she wrote, "Tomorrow will be Sacrament Sunday, I have read over all my history, a history of miserable woe, mistakes and blinding vanity, of seeking great things for myself." The theme was repeated over and over again in her private writings, reflecting the conflict between "doing for myself" and "doing for others in God's name." As a career, nursing was admirably suited to control and direct this conflict, even though it did not remove it—indeed, to remove it would have been to remove the driving force itself. By choosing nursing, with all of its outer-directed and masochistic implications, she could absorb her fury, satisfy her drive for power, and at the same time placate the demands of her extremely strong superego by directing her efforts to the aid of others "in God's name." The need for power was itself rooted in her conflict with her mother and sister, which influenced every stage of her psychosocial and psychosexual development.

Florence Nightingale's career choice was not primarily directed toward producing pleasure by providing a channel for the unconscious investment of libidinal and aggressive emotional energy. "My work: an idol, a Molloch to me," she wrote in 1877 in another oft-repeated sentiment. Rather than a source of pleasure, her work was more a shield against discomfort, an external support to her defenses, which helped to control internal conflict and anxiety by deflecting energy from fantasy to action. Her attempts to control the basic conflict that permeated her personality and stymied her effort to find a niche in society were successful only at great emotional cost in each of the stages of her life cycle, but one doubts that the happy old woman would have chosen any other way.

It should be obvious to the reader that this article represents but the first leg of a long journey on the road to a full understanding of the psychological forces that permitted Florence Nightingale to achieve such extraordinary power and influence. In this study we have relied chiefly on the signposts set out by Freud, Erikson, and Deutsch, i.e., the oedipal approach, which has been extremely useful in pointing the way. In the stages that lie ahead, however, other road maps will have to be used. Since, for example, in this first investigation a severely vulnerable narcissism has emerged as a primary characteristic of Florence Nightingale's personality, it will be necessary to apply the newer theories of narcissism such as are found in the works of Kohut.

Some of the way can already be charted. Florence Nightingale had a strong need for revenge, for righting wrongs, for undoing a hurt by whatever means, and an unrelenting compulsion to pursue these aims until she was able to blot out the offense against her. The matrix of her narcissistic rage is probably to be found in her sense of abandonment. Her traumatic reactions as a child when "abandoned" by the females to whom she had been passionately attached—such as her nurse, Miss Christie, or Aunt Mai—coupled with her reactions all through life to any hint of desertion and her lack of empathy toward the offender lead one to surmise that she blamed her family, and particularly her mother, first for abandoning her to her nurse, and second for the subsequent desertions by the nurse and other females to whom she became attached. Nobody else would ever be able to come so close to her, including her unsuccessful suitors. She could therefore protect herself against further abandonment while at the same time use the weapon that she so feared against others. Thus, with anything even remotely resembling desertion, as when Aunt Mai quite naturally returned to her family after years of sacrifice to Florence, her rage was unbounded and irrational. The degree which such rage could reach is best seen in her remarkable reaction to Sidney Herbert's death—she blamed Herbert and God for Herbert's "desertion" of her. Only in old age was this narcissistic anger blunted because all of those who could injure her by abandonment were dead. Thus, her shame subsided, and with it, her rage.

Future research on a psychohistorical study of Florence Nightingale will have to include not only the best observations emanating from psychoanalysis but also new information on her pregenital and adolescent development, which has not yet come to light either in the previously published biographies or in the main corpus of her own writings and papers. Only then will we be able to present a complete psychohistorical interpretation of this fascinating, and captivating woman.

Florence Nightingale
and the Crimean War:
The "Lady with a Lamp"
Saint? Heroine?

The Reverend Sidney Godolphin Osborne, a well-known nineteenth century philanthropist and friend of Secretary at War Sidney Herbert had arbitrarily and uninvited, gone to Scutari as a volunteer chaplain. Seeking the truth on this self-imposed mission he determined, "whether that truth would please or displease the public, or the Government, was to me a matter of indifference; I had nothing to gain or to fear from either." While in Scutari he made an unofficial inspection of all hospitals under Florence Nightingale's care. The results, not unlike the many reports sent back to England by *London Times* correspondent William Howard Russell, were published in a book entitled *Scutari and its Hospitals* (1855). In these excerpts from the Preface and Chapters IV and V, can be found an account of the general conditions as well as many of the scenes he experienced. The book caused much consternation among the leaders responsible for the war's blunders but, while vividly pointing these out, it also assesses how the hospitals would have totally collapsed if Miss Nightingale had not been present.

SIDNEY GODOLPHIN OSBORNE (1808-1889)

An Eye-Witness Account

PREFACE

In the following pages I am afraid my readers will find little that can afford pleasure. If I had aimed at writing on this unhappy subject that which would have pleased, I must have aimed also to deceive. I can claim this much for myself, the facts I relate, the opinions I have given, are from an independent witness. I went upon my self-imposed mission, altogether unfettered, I had nothing to gain from any one particular course of conduct. I sought the truth, and took my own way to arrive at it. Whether that truth would please or displease the public, or the Government, was to me a matter of indifference; I had nothing to gain or to fear from either.

I have in my possession ample means of proving, that I did press upon the Authorities in the East, and at home, the existence of that shameful state of things I now thus publish; and that on my return home, I did receive the thanks of the Government, for my efforts at Scutari.

Since the greater part of this volume was prepared for the press, the force of public opinion has exacted from the "executive," a Parliamentary Committee of Enquiry; I rejoice at this, if only as a small instalment of the justice that should be done, to the memory of the many thousands of my fellow creatures, who I believe, lost their lives through the apathy, ignorance, folly and misconduct of the parties immediately entrusted with the details of this war.

That this Committee will ever get at to expose, those who have been the most culpable, I do not believe; for I know well how easy it is for powerful popular men in high station, to so trammell these enquiries, as to shield the great offenders, and sacrifice the subalterns. I know in this case, there has already been a disposition, to try by the sacrifice of one nobleman, to turn the tide of public curiosity from too narrow a scrutiny of the conduct of those, who were just as responsible as he was, but who had not the manliness to admit it.

In my own opinion the whole of the Cabinet of which the Duke of Newcastle was a member, were quite as open to accusation as he was. The most culpable of all, was that very noble Lord, who stamping the affairs of the East as "horrible and heartrending," still sat at the table with the Minister at War, until it served his purpose to make a merit of his betrayal.

"Horrible, heartrending" as has been the Camp and Scutari records of the war; reflecting as they do most justly on the Commander-in-Chief, whose apathy seems to have blinded him to them, and on the officials at home and abroad whose blundering carelessness worked such horrors. The country seems to me to have suffered still greater humiliation from the conduct of its rulers, in their endeavor to evade enquiry and shield the true culprits.

This nation has paid a fearful penalty in "life" for the mis-management of the war. When the pressure of the cost in "means" is fully felt, I hope the spirit of the land may be roused, to require at the hands of those who rule these matters, that for the future, the lives of our soldiers, the hard-earned money of the tax-payers, shall not be wantonly made over to the wasteful expenditure of men; who neither in the Cabinet, the field, or in any one department, have proved that they possess either administrative power, or common sense habits of business. . . .

IV

I must now conduct my readers to another part of the Barrack Hospital, and one most interesting. On entering by the gate at the "main guard," turning directly to the left, at a short distance there is a wooden partition across a corridor; passing through the door in this you come to one of the usual lanes hedged in by the beds of the wounded; at its furthest extremity is the tower, in which the "sisters" have their "quarters." Whatever of neglect may attach elsewhere, none can be imputed here. From this tower flowed that well directed stream of untiring benevolence and charitable exertion, which has been deservedly the theme of so much praise. Here there has been no idleness, no standing still, no waiting for orders from home, no quibbling with any requisition made upon those, who so cheerfully administered the stores at their disposal.

Entering the door leading into the "sisters" tower, you at once found yourself a spectator of a busy and most interesting scene. There is a large room, with two or three doors opening from it on one side; on the other, one door opening into an apartment in which many of the Nurses and Sisters slept, and had I believe their meals. In the centre was a large kitchen table; bustling about this, might be seen the High Priestess of the room Mrs. C——; often as I have had occasion to pass through this room, I do not ever recollect finding her either absent from it, or unoccupied.

At this table she received the various matters from the kitchen and stores of the Sisterhood, which attendant Sisters or Nurses were ever ready to take to the sick in any and every part of these gigantic hospitals. It was a curious scene, and a close study of it afforded a practical lesson in the working of true common sense benevolence. There were constant fresh arrivals of various matters ready either for immediate distribution, or for preparation for it; there was also as frequent an arrival of requisitions for some of the many good things, over which Mrs. C—— presided with intiring perseverance.

The floor on one side of the room, was loaded with packages of all kinds, stores of things for the internal and external consumption of the patients; bales of shirts, socks, slippers, dressing gowns, flannel; heaps of every sort of article, likely to be of use in affording comfort and securing cleanliness. It gave one some idea of what such a room would be in a good hospital, if on some sudden alarm, it had been made a place of refuge for articles snatched from its every store. In reality it was one feature of a bold attempt upon the part of extraneous benevolence, to supply the deficiencies of the various departments, which as a matter of course should have supplied all these things. On the right hand side of the room, were doors leading to the private room of Miss Nightingale, and to the dormitories of the Nuns, and their Reverend Mother, a lady of whom all spoke in the highest terms.

In the further corner of the right hand side, was the entrance to the sitting room occupied by Miss Nightingale and her friends the Bracebridges. I shall ever recall with the liveliest satisfaction, the many visits I paid to this apartment. Here were held those councils over which Miss Nightingale so ably presided, at which were discussed the measures necessary to meet the daily varying exigencies of the hospitals. From hence were given the orders which regulated the female staff, working under this most gifted Head. This too was the office from which were sent those many letters to the government, to friends and supporters at home, which told such awful tales of the sufferings of the sick and wounded, their utter want of so many necessaries. Here might be seen the "Times" almoner, taking down in his note book from day to day, the list of things he was pressed to obtain, which might all with a little activity have been provided as easily by the authorities of the hospital.

To attempt the narration of the business transacted in this room, would be a task beyond my powers. It was of a nature comprehending somewhat of the detail of every recognized "department;" it embraced the consideration of every failure of duty on the part of "authorities" at home and on the spot; it aimed at the attainment of order and humanity by limited means, to be directed against the widest possible field of disorganization.

Had Miss Nightingale and her Staff taken up their post in the best regulated hospital conceivable, with four thousand patients, their task would have taxed to the utmost their every energy. Here was an utter want of all regulation, it was a mere unseemly scramble; the Staff was altogether deficient in strength; the commissariat and purveying department, as weak in power as in capacity; there was no real Head, and there existed on all sides a state of feeling, which was inclined to resent all non-military interference; whilst at the same time, it was shamefully obvious that there was no one feature of military order. Jealous of each other, jealous of every one else, with some few bright exceptions, there was little encouragement from any of the officials, for any one out of mere benevolence to lend any aid. The fact is, the stout denial of the shameful condition of the hospitals, made to the authorities at home, could not be made on the spot, the officials therefore walked about self-convicted. As a warm friend of the government, sent out under the direct sanction of the War Office, I am satisfied it was the wish of Miss Nightingale to make the best of everything. She at once found the real truth, and cheerfully and gratefully availed herself of that help from irregular sources, which to this moment has been her chief support.

My readers will very naturally expect that I should give them some particulars regarding this lady. I can only give the result of my own observation and experience; for on such a matter, I should be sorry to draw for my information from other sources. Miss Nightingale in appearance, is just what you would expect in any other well-bred woman, who may have seen perhaps rather more than thirty years of life; her manner and countenance are prepossessing, and this without the possession of positive beauty; it is a face not easily forgotten, pleasing in its smile, with an eye betokening great self possession, and giving when she wishes, a quiet look of firm determination to every feature. Her general demeanour is quiet and rather reserved; still I am much mistaken if she is not gifted with a very lively sense of the ridiculous. In conversation, she speaks on matters of business with a grave earnestness, one would not expect from her appearance. She has evidently a mind disciplined to restrain under the principles of the action of the moment, every feeling which would interfere with it. She has trained herself to command, and learned the value of conciliation towards others, and constraint over herself. I can conceive her to be a strict disciplinarian; she throws herself into a work—as its Head—as such she knows well how much success must depend upon literal obedience to her every order. She seems to understand business thoroughly, though to me she had the failure common to many "Heads," a too great love of management in the small details which had better perhaps have been left to others. Her nerve is wonderful; I have been with her at very severe operations; she was more than equal to the trial. She has an utter disregard of contagion; I have known her spend hours over men dying of cholera or fever. The more awful to every sense any particular case, especially if it was that of a dying man, her slight form would be seen bending over him, administering to his ease in every way in her power, and seldom quitting his side till death released him.

I have heard and read with indignation, the remarks hazarded upon her religious character. I found her myself to be in her every word and action a Christian; I thought this quite enough. It would have been in my opinion the most cruel impertinence, to scrutinize her words and acts, to discover to which of the many bodies of true Christians she belonged. I have conversed with her several times on the deaths of those, who I had visited ministerially in the hospitals, with whom she had been when they died. I never heard one word from her lips, that would not have been just what I should have expected from the lips of those who I have known to be the most experienced and devout of our common faith. Her work ought to answer for her faith; at least none should dare to call that faith in question, in opposition to such work, on grounds so weak and trivial as those I have seen urged. That she has been equally kind and attentive to men of every creed; that she would smooth the pillow and give water to a dying fellow creature who might own no creed, I have no doubt; all honour to her that she does feel, that her's is the Samaritan's—not the Pharisee's work. If there is blame in looking for a Roman Catholic priest to attend a dying Romanist, let me share it with her—I did it again and again.

Those who walked that field of suffering, had too many pressing calls on every energy which could be enlisted to save pain to the body, to stop to question the faith of the sufferers. It was not the least frightful of the many features of that awful scene, that the demand for active physical help, did sadly interfere with the aid which would have been cheerfully given in higher matters. We all did what we could in both; but this was a hospital, Miss Nightingale and her staff were nurses, cooks, purveyors; they were not, they could not be, but in a very minor degree—missionaries. Although to the last, I myself gladly seized every opportunity of praying with, or reading to any dying man, I was soon obliged to give up devoting myself to that work, for I felt that this could be done by others; there was a daily increasing demand upon me in some other important matters, which few beside myself, from circumstances, could have undertaken.

I do not think it is possible to measure the real difficulties of the work Miss Nightingale has done, and is doing, by the mere magnitude of the field, and its peculiarly horrible nature. Every day brought some new complication of misery, to be somehow unravelled by the power ruling in the sisters' tower. Each day had its peculiar trial to one who had taken such a load of responsibility, in an untried field, and with a staff of her own sex, all new to it. Her's was a post requiring the courage of a Cardigan, the tact and diplomacy of a Palmerston, the endurance of a Howard, the cheerful philanthropy of a Mrs. Fry or a Miss Neave; Miss Nightingale yet fills that post, and in my opinion is the one individual, who in this whole unhappy war, has shown more than any other, what real energy guided by good sense can do, to meet the calls of sudden emergency.

There must have been when I left Scutari little less than four miles of ground occupied in lines of beds; the reader may from this conceive the pressure upon the physical and mental powers of the sisters. That many of them proved unequal to the work was to be expected; the wonder to me is, how any have survived it. Many ought never to have entered upon it. A hospital of this sort in the offices it demands from the nurses—and all the sisterhood may be considered as nurses—in the scenes with which it surrounds them, makes no ordinary demand on the female mind. It is an hourly endurance in a distant country, of trials to many a sense, which at home would scarce seem endurable for a moment.

This is no such nursing as that afforded in the rooms of the sick at home, be they our relatives or friends, or those of our poorer fellow creatures. We all know, at least the most of us alas! do, what it is to watch around the sick beds of friends and relatives. We know how the exigencies of a sick room break through all the mere conventionalities of every day life. Where all have their every interest for the time absorbed in the endeavour to minister to the comfort of the sick one by whom they watch; where friends, relatives, and servants have this one object in view—real delicacy consists in being insensible to every thing else. When even in distant passages, they who meet speak in whispers, in the actual room of apprehended death, the very atmosphere of the scene makes all things as pure, as the motives that call for the sympathy and aid afforded.

This is very different in the case of such a scene of death and suffering as that at Scutari. The nurse or sister nursing, is hurried from one spot of a vast scene of death to another; at each successive bed to which she may be summoned, she has to minister to one a stranger to her. Surrounded as she is by masses only differing in the nature, but little in the degree of suffering, it is impossible for her so to centre her whole mind upon any one case, as to acquire that perfect command over the delicacy of feeling, to which English women are bred, attainable in an ordinary sick room. The trials to which Miss Nightingale as the head of the sisterhood is exposed, are so far greater than those of the other sisters, in that she has a greater weight of responsibility; but there is not one of that devoted band, who does not each day pass an ordeal to her every womanly sense, beyond all description. The dressing the wounds of the men, the attendance upon those who are in the agonies of death, is but a small part of the field of duty, on which these ladies have so boldly entered.

In my own opinion it would be most advisable that the hired professional nurses, should wear some dress distinguishing them from the sisters. There are many offices about the sick and wounded which the surgeons would at once require, and with reason, of a hired hospital nurse, which nothing could induce them to ask of a "sister." I am also quite satisfied this is no field of usefulness proper for young English women. We are very apt to confound the duties and the office of these volunteer ladies, with those of the sisters of charity in the French hospitals. From what I saw and could learn at those hospitals, the several positions in life of the respective parties; their training, the obligation of the religious vow, &c.—make a very wide distinction between them.

England and the English Army will ever owe a deep debt of gratitude to the Ladies who have devoted themselves to this first attempt, to introduce the zeal and tender care of well-bred women, into the economy of a Military Hospital. When the war is over, and they return to us, from their experience may be gained the valuable information, how far all the work they had to do in this crisis, was work that in the sober moment of calm consideration at home, they would recommend as a field for the charitable exertion of English ladies. I have little doubt but the majority would agree with me, that very much of it had been better left, had it been possible, to trained paid nurses; and that there would have still remained a large field of more fitting usefulness for the zeal of unpaid volunteers.

A good deal I know has been said in public, and in private about the prevalence throughout the Protestant part of the Sisterhood, of what are called Puseyite principles. It was a matter into which I did not seek to enquire; it was sufficient for me to see that on whatever Church principles it was done, true charity was never better represented; it was a field leaving no room, affording no leisure for any outbreak of those polemical bitternesses, which so poison the atmosphere of our common christianity at home. Those ladies I had most to do with when taking Chaplain duty were from Miss Sellon's Sisterhood. I found them most active in finding out for me every case in their district where I could render any service. There may have been jealousies and religious (?) heartburnings; where is the spot on which they do not exist? I never saw anything of it myself, all worked as of one mind.

I must not pass over my friends Mr. and Mrs. Bracebridge; the latter ever watchful over her charge Miss Nightingale, was most useful to her; indeed without such a Motherly friend, I cannot see how she could have got through many of the trials of her position. Mr. Bracebridge was active everywhere, and from his acquaintance with the East, his persevering good humoured attempts to help every-body about everything, was of infinite service. Hitherto God has been most merciful in supporting the Sisters and Nurses, in their work of true christian love. It is impossible to magnify the amount of labour they undertake. They will have their reward at that day when the Great Preacher to the quick and dead, shall practically prove the weight and truth of the text.—"I was sick and ye visited me."

V

I have hitherto spoken of the sick and wounded soldiers as I saw them within the walls of the Hospitals. To an ordinary observer a few weeks after the battle of Inkermann, the corridors of these buildings however painful the sight they presented, would have given a very favourable view of the general condition of the sick and wounded compared with what it had been, and still was in some particulars. I have spoken strongly on the subject of the internal economy of these Hospitals; there were features connected with their external economy, of which it is impossible to speak in adequate terms of indignation and disgust. If the sick and wounded soldier did get at last fair and humane treatment when within the Hospital walls at Scutari, it was I firmly believe owing to the efforts of those who had no official position there. Who can describe what they had to suffer on board the transport ships on their way to Scutari, and in the transit from those ships to the Hospitals?

I made a practice of frequently going down to the pier to assist at the landing of these poor creatures; for I not only found I could thus myself render service, but I found also, that from some cause or other, my being present seemed to act beneficially in securing more humanity from the attendant officials. To the day on which I left, there was not only a very great want of stretchers on which to carry the wounded, but there was not one single covered stretcher—all were of the very roughest construction. The bearers were invalid soldiers for the most part unequal to the work, Turkish soldiers, stupid, careless, and unfeeling, and for a time a gang of porters from Constantinople wholly unused to bear any weight in an upright position, and therefore very ill adapted for the purpose.

It is now a matter beyond all contradiction that the way in which the sick and wounded were brought from Balaklava to Scutari, was in its every detail utterly indefensible. They were put on board in a condition demanding the utmost care; many had fresh severe wounds, some had undergone recent amputation, many were weak to the last degree, the generality of their clothing wholly insufficient; and yet they were crowded together between and sometimes on the decks, with not even an apology for a bed; some, indeed I fear many of them, were even without a blanket to lie on.

As to any nursing, as the rule all they could expect was, that which some eight or ten invalid soldiers could afford; on these men, the sea and the smell from the crowded decks produced such an effect, that they were themselves soon added to the list of sick. The medical assistance was altogether inadequate; in some cases it can scarce have been said to have existed at all. The medicines and medical comforts, were either altogether wanting, or only put on board in such quantities, as to be a mere mockery.

The only food some 200 or more wretched suffering and sick men had afforded to them, was the usual salt rations of ship diet, and this many of them could not eat; in some of the ships the water was so stored that the weakest men could not get at it, and had no one to get it for them. The Mauritius brought down a large number of these poor creatures, and so shamefully had the authorities provided for them, in so awful a condition were they, that a Colonel of one of the regiments, himself wounded, who came with them told me, that if it had not been for the exertions of the civil Surgeon and the sailors belonging to the transport ship, with some soldier's wives, many must have died from positive neglect; I thought the conduct of these sailors and women to be in such striking contrast to that of the authorities, that I went on board and distributed ten pounds amongst them.

From some government returns I have in my possession, it is made to appear as if the average voyage from Balaklava to Scutari was four days and a half. This is to me a tampering with the truth; it may have been the average passage between the two places, but vessels have been fourteen days with sick on board before they left the Crimea, another week after anchoring in the Bosphorus, before the sick were landed. I have known passengers coming down in these ships, obliged to leave them from the dreadful stench proceeding from between decks where the sick were huddled together. As to any of the conveniences necessary for men who could not stir from where they were placed, they never seem to have been thought of. Individuals of respectability who have made the voyage in these vessels when thus freighted, have declared to me, that the dreadful cruelty of the whole treatment of these poor men was beyond all belief—it has been well called "the middle passage."

The Officers who came down to the Bosphorus with the Avon, will I think never forget the horrors they witnessed; I have been furnished with some details of that passage, and also of the voyages of other transports; they are too dreadful for publication; of course many died under this system of barbarous neglect; those who survived were landed in a condition so miserable, that one could scarcely have congratulated them on their escape.

I will give an instance of how this painful treatment of the sick and wounded was sometimes needlessly prolonged. The Medway had

had her melancholy freight on board nearly three weeks; she was anchored less than a quarter of a mile from Scutari. I went over early one morning in hopes of aiding in moving the poor creatures to the hospital on shore. As I crossed the Bosphorus, I met the large boats we usually employed for the purpose, going over to the Golden Horn loaded with soldiers returning to the Crimea; when I reached Scutari pier, I found the authorities energetically abusing Admiral Boxer, who had thus taken possession of the only boats by which the sick could be landed; the consequence was, the day was lost, and we had for the three next days weather which defied any attempt to bring them ashore. I have in another chapter endeavoured to give some idea of the inconvenience of the landing place at Scutari, and the scene of confusion it presented. The large boats bringing the sick and wounded ashore, came alongside the only sound part of this so-called pier. Those who were very severely wounded were brought on stretchers; they had then to be lifted out and placed on the ground; four men were called from the crowd of invalid orderlies marched down for the purpose; the stretcher was then lifted on to their shoulders, and they started to face the steep long ascent with their melancholy burden. These bearers were not only often so physically weak as to be unfit for the work, but no one seemed disposed to take any pains to choose men of equal height for any one stretcher. The groans of the poor creatures thus carried were often most painful to hear. Occasionally there were not bearers enough, and I have seen the wounded men lying for some considerable length of time on the damp surface of the pier, waiting till more came. When the poor fellows had been thus carried to the hospital, they were sometimes subjected to still further painful trial, being put down and taken up again and again, before the authorities could determine in what part of the hospital they were to be placed.

I must say this wanton addition to suffering, was not confined to the cases of common soldiers; more than one officer has known something of it in his own person. It will hardly be believed, but it cannot be denied, that men almost in the last hours of their existence have been carried up to the barrack hospital, sent on from thence the rough half mile to the general hospital, and then sent back again, because there was no room for them.

When I recollect how the poor wounded men of the Balaklava and Inkermann actions, groaned with pain even when lifted from the boats with the greatest care; when I call to mind how from the evident nature of some of their wounds, any, the least motion must have been most painful; all the indignation I felt at the time, returns upon me at

the utter want of feeling, with which their transport from the ships
to the hospital was effected. I could well enter into the feelings of
one officer who himself lying wounded on a stretcher, seemed so disgusted with the whole scene, that he exclaimed,"do cover my face for
me;" it was indeed a trial of any man's nerves, to see the way this
important part of the public service was misconducted.

Let the reader now imagine himself standing on the highest part
of the paved acclivity, leading from Scutari pier to the Barrack Hospital, at a time when the sick and wounded were being landed from one
of these transport ships. A procession would pass him of perhaps the
most melancholy character it is possible to conceive. One after another
in quick succession would be seen groups of four weak, ill clad, pale,
weary invalids—(they called them convalescents), staggering up the
ascent with a stretcher on their shoulders bearing one of England's
heroes; many of them in the very clothes in which they fought, never
having had more than just enough of them removed, to enable the
surgeons to dress their wounds or amputate their limbs. Their ghastly
appearance, the evident famine as well as pain stamped upon their
countenance, told it's own sad tale; the stretchers were so badly constructed, the bearers so little equal to the task, that the poor men thus
carried, were for ever crying out with agony at each change of their
position, caused by the difficulty with which they could be carried at
all, by such weak men, over such difficult ground. For hours with
little interruption would this file of bearers with their living load pass
by you.

It was hard to conceive anything more piteous than this, and yet
from time to time, in slower but yet in too quick succession, other
objects even more pitiable would come under view. Far too great a
number of these unfortunate men were obliged to walk from the pier
to the hospital, some even without that support afforded by one or
more orderlies, which others were so fortunate as to obtain. Very many
of them were mere spectres; they did in reality more belong to the dead
than to the living, for death was stamped indelibly upon them. They
could, even when helped, scarcely crawl over this rough, hard, steep
road; and let me add, that they frequently had been more than six
hours without any food. I am told that a certain Member of Parliament
was so shocked at one of these cases, that he actually carried the man
himself. I have given them often sherry, and brandy and water which
I took with me for the purpose, and it seemed as though they scarcely
had the power to swallow it. It will not be denied, that many of these
poor creatures had thus to walk, because there was not a sufficient

number of stretchers to carry them, or if there had been, of orderlies to carry the stretchers. So weak were some of these bearers, that on one occasion, when I had to land and convey a friend, an officer wounded at Inkermann, from the farthest pier to the General Hospital, one of them was so faint, I had to get rid of him and replace him by a soldier passing at the time.

But will it be believed that after these poor sinking, sick, and wounded men had made their painful journey to the Barrack Hospital from the Scutari pier, I have seen them, walked up and down the wards, whilst a distracted official was in vain trying to find them beds. I have known them to be left on one occasion for a length of time huddled together in a ward without beds, and even in the open yard exposed to heavy rain: this was the case with the sick from the "Gertrude" but a few days before I left. It is no matter of surprise to me, that there were deaths between the ship's side and the hospital.

And what a scene was it to see them stripped and washed! I can stand by an unmoved spectator of any the severest operation; I have in the East and elsewhere seen such destruction of the human frame, by disease, fire or violence, as at the time almost to destroy any power I had of rendering assistance, so sickened have I been; but I have never seen worked out upon the human body anything so truly horrifying, as was shown upon the naked frames of these men. I know, for I studied it in Ireland, the well-defined characteristics of famine; it is a matter in which I do not think I can be deceived, for starvation can be recognized by a practised eye, quite as easily as many of the diseases we are subject to which are unmistakeable. It is my belief that a very large proportion of these so called sick, were men who *had been starved.* The food served to them in the camp was not sufficient, had they been ever so well sheltered; there were other bad features in it besides that poisonous one the green coffee. The way the men were worked, and not sheltered, whilst it exposed them to utter exhaustion of physical power, often forbad them getting at their wretched ill-cooked rations, until they were so sick they could not touch them. They literally *fell* sick, were put on board the transports, in the condition I have spoken of above; on board these ships, these famine stricken men, had no other rations than salt meat and hard ship biscuit. In rare instances I could trace out the fact of some rice having been served out a few times on the voyage.

I fully expect much of what I have here written will be strenuously denied; on the evidence of my own eyes, on the testimony of upright impartial witnesses, I am prepared to assert, I have given a very modified, rather than a high coloured view of what this transport service, and the system pursued in landing the sick, really was. I challenged the attention of the Commissioners sent out by the Duke of Newcastle, to it at the time, on the spot, in terms which left them no room for doubt, that in my opinion nothing could be more disgraceful, more wantonly cruel; I reported it to Lord Redcliffe, and sent a letter direct to the Minister of War on the subject. I have reason to know that even to this day, the improvement has been far more a matter of promise than of reality.

I would have my readers bear in mind, that many of these poor suffering ill-treated men, were from the ranks of "the Guards" whose departure for the East caused such a sensation in London. I wish the Queen could have seen them, when after having won all the glory for her army, that the most sanguine of their admirers could have hoped for, they met that sad, cruel treatment, which all would have considered common humanity, the commonest foresight, might have spared them. I well remember the feeling with which I read the account of their march through the streets of London, and their embarkation; I felt as I read it how natural were the tears of many of the spectators, the excitement of all who looked on that noble body of men, the very flower of our army, the men on whom the nation knew it could depend for deeds of bravery, worthy of their of old well earned fame.

Are we to forget, or lightly forgive the treatment to which these and others as brave of our soldiers were so wantonly exposed? In my opinion, neither in the triumph of victory, if we are yet so blessed, or in the shame and degradation of defeat, if defeat with shame can by possibility be contemplated, should this nation forget, that it is its bounden duty to trace out how, by whose negligence, by whose ignorance it happened, that men whose deeds of heroism we were swift to acknowledge in the field, when wounded and sick, were subject to such want of the commonest care and humanity. There is the greater claim in this matter for enquiry, as I am satisfied, the government at home had taken considerable pains to order the very necessaries the want of which was most felt; and had empowered the English Ambassador on the spot, to meet promptly without regard to expense, every requisition made to him. It must have been clear to the dullest in capacity of the officials at Scutari, that a great deal of what I have now described, might have been provided against, by a very little activity, and a very small outlay of money. With regard to the astounding list of necessary stores, I here record my solemn conviction, that in this matter, there must have been something worse than negligence on the part of the departments at home. I cannot believe they were all shipped for the East; for it is to me wholly impossible that such a bulk of goods could be even in the East mis-laid. I can from what I have learned lately of the way in which public business is conducted, far more easily come to the conclusion, that the discovery of these stores would be more properly put into the hands of my friend Sir Richard Mayne, than into that of any "commission."

As to the way the sick were treated at Balaklava, were put on board ship, and the ships ordered to sail unfound in attendance, in food, and in the necessaries common decency demanded, I for one cannot remove the weight of this national disgrace, from the door of the Commander in Chief and his Staff. The facts could not have been kept from him, had he been commonly active himself, or been served by a staff disposed to do its duty. It would be to me a betrayal of all justice, treason to every christian feeling, if I did not thus state what I believe to be the truth. There are plenty of pens and voices to defend Generals and Staff Officers; they can speak and write for themselves; my poor clients if living dare not speak; but alas! how few have been spared to prove that power of endurance, which will so suffer, and yet not complain.

This excerpt from a book entitled *Heroines of Modern Progress* provides a sample of the popular view of Florence Nightingale—the "Angel of the Crimea" with its heavy emphasis on her Crimean War exploits. While presenting a series of "intimate character sketches of women in their proper social and historical setting," the stated purpose of the entire work is to show "how they reacted upon society in a way that, while still personal, touched so great and general a need that they became representatives of millions, and hence leaders, truly heroines of modern progress". Written for the general reader, without footnotes, this romanticized portrait is similar to many like it that appeared in the 1930's. Summarizing her accomplishments in the Crimea, for example, the authors said:

> She conquered disease. And it is not too much to say that she conquered the Russian army, and saved the war for the allies. No wonder England welcomed her home as one of the greatest heroines in all her history.

ELMER C. ADAMS and WARREN DUNHAM FOSTER

"Heroine of Modern Progress"

. . . The Crimean war was in progress, France and England being allied to defend Turkey against Russian aggression. The British army had sailed to a strange climate with shamefully poor commissary and medical staffs. The weather was stormy and the soldiers had little shelter against it. Said a correspondent of the *London Times,* "It is now pouring rain, the skies are black as ink, the wind is howling over the staggering tents, the trenches are turned into dykes; in the tents the water is sometimes a foot deep; our men have not either warm or waterproof clothing; they are out for twelve hours at a time in the trenches"—and so on without end.

Plenty of food and clothing had been shipped from England, but they never reached their destination. Some vessels were delayed; in some the stores were packed at the bottom of the hold and could not be raised; some hove in with the wrong goods at the wrong port— and, on one, the consignment of boots proved to be all for the left foot! But the most criminal point of mismanagement was this: food, clothing and medicine might be stored in a warehouse within easy reach of the army; but the official with authority to deal them out would be absent, and, so stringent were the army rules that no one dared so much as point at them! The rigid system was infinitely worse than no system. And the soldiers were starving in the midst of plenty, and freezing under the shadow of mountains of good woolen clothing.

Now, to come at once to the worst, imagine these conditions transferred to the military hospitals. In the great Barrack Hospital at Scutari lay two thousand sorely wounded men, and hundreds more were coming in every day. The wards were crowded to twice their capacity—the sick lay side by side on mattresses that touched each other. The floors and walls and ceilings were wet and filthy. There was no ventilation. Rats and vermin swarmed everywhere. The men lay "in their uniforms, stiff with gore and covered with filth to a degree and of a kind no one could write about." It was a "dreadful den of dirt, pestilence and death."

This might have been remedied by an adequate medical staff. But the doctors were few. They were hampered in their professional duties by administrative ones. And they had to trust the actual nursing to orderlies who had never seen sickness in their lives. Then, there was the same lack of supplies due to mismanagement. There "were no vessels for water or utensils of any kind; no soap, towels or cloths, no hospital clothes." "The sheets were of canvas and so coarse that the wounded men begged to be left in their blankets. There was no bed-room furniture of any kind, and only beer or wine bottles for candle-sticks!" It is difficult to imagine a scene of worse disorder and misery. The proportion of deaths to the whole army, from disease alone—malaria and cholera—was sixty per cent. Seventy died in the hospital in one night. There was danger that the entire army would be wiped out,—most of it without ever receiving a scratch from the enemy's weapons.

It was in this extremity that the British nation appealed to Florence Nightingale to save the sick and wounded men,—an army of twenty-eight thousand as helpless as children before the ravages of disease—and to save the war. Was ever a bigger task put upon a woman?

And was ever a bigger honor? Female nurses had never before been admitted to English military hospitals, because English nurses anywhere had been something of a nuisance. This woman must have proved that she was not a nuisance. For the minister of war requested her to organize a band of nurses for Scutari and gave her power to draw upon the government to any extent.

Miss Nightingale at the time was thirty-four years old. An acquaintance described her thus: "Simple, intellectual, sweet, full of love and benevolence, she is a fascinating and perfect woman. She is tall and pale. Her face is exceedingly lovely. But better than all is the soul's glory that shines through every feature so exultingly. Nothing can be sweeter than her smile. It is like a sunny day in summer." Again, "young, (about the age of our Queen) graceful, feminine, rich, popular, she holds a singularly gentle and persuasive influence over all with whom she comes in contact. Her friends and acquaintances are of all classes and persuasions, but her happiest place is at home in the center of a very large band of accomplished relatives, and in simplest obedience to her admiring parents."

Nevertheless Scutari needed her. She was ready for Scutari. It was that for which she had been unconsciously preparing since a girl. She was ready, and she went.

Within six days from the time she accepted the post, Miss Nightingale had selected thirty-eight nurses, and departed for the seat of war. She arrived at Scutari November 4, 1854, and walked the length of the barracks, viewing her two miles of patients. And next day before she could form any plans, the fresh victims of another battle began to arrive. There was not space for them within the walls and hundreds had to repose, with what comfort they could, in the mud outside. One of the nurses wrote, "Many died immediately after being brought in—their moans would pierce the heart—and the look of agony on those poor dying faces will never leave my heart." A terrible situation to face; and all England depending on her!

But the nurse did not hesitate. She ordered the patients brought in, and directed where to lay them, and what attention they should have. She was up and around twenty hours that day, and as many the next, until a place had been found for every man, even in the corridors and on the landings of the stair. As leader of the nurses she might have confined herself to administrative tasks—of which there were enough for any woman—and stayed in the office. But no. She shrank from the sight of no operation. Many men, indeed, whose cases the surgeons thought hopeless, she nursed back to health. A visitor saw her one morning at two o'clock at the bedside of a dying soldier, lamp in hand. She was writing down his last message to the home folks; and for them, too, she took in charge his watch and trinkets—and then soothed him in his last moments. And this was but one case in thousands. "She is a ministering angel, without any exaggeration, in these hospitals," wrote a correspondent of the *London Times*, "and as the slender form glides quietly along each corridor, every poor fellow's face softens with gratitude at the sight of her. When all the medical officers have retired for the night, and silence and darkness have settled down upon the miles of prostrate sick, she may be observed alone, with lamp in hand, making her solitary rounds."

One soldier said, "I can't help crying when I see them. Only think of Englishwomen coming out here to nurse us; it is so homely and comfortable." He probably did not cry alone. And one wrote to his people, "She would speak to one and another and nod and smile to many more; but she could not do it to all, you know, for we lay there by hundreds; but we could kiss her shadow as it fell, and lay our heads on our pillows again content!" It was of this incident that Longfellow wrote in his "Lady with the lamp":

> And slow, as in a dream of bliss,
> The speechless sufferer turns to kiss
> Her shadow as it falls
> Upon the darkening walls.

In a place like Scutari, however, this kind of feminine tenderness alone would avail little. Science was needed; the most perfect skill in scientific nursing. The windows were few, and the few were mostly locked; and where one was opened the odors of decaying animals came in to pollute still more the foul air of the wards.

The food for the whole hospital—for those sick of fever, cholera, wounds and what not, as well as for those in health—was cooked, like and "Irish stew," in big kettles. Vegetables and meats were dumped in together, and when any one felt hungry he could dip for himself. Naturally some got food overdone, and some got it raw; the luckiest got a mess that was scarcely palatable; and the sick could generally not eat at all. As for other matters, it has been shown how unclean the barrack wards were, how "only seven shirts" had been laundered in all those wretched weeks, and how the infected bed linen of all classes of patients was thrown, unsorted into one general wash.

But Florence Nightingale had spent twelve years in the hospitals of Europe to learn how to conquer just such situations as this. She had the waste and pollution outside the walls cleared away. Then she threw up the windows, and set a carpenter to make more. Within ten days she had established a diet kitchen and was feeding the men each on the food his particular case demanded. She set up a laundry, too, where the garments of the sick could be cleansed in a sanitary way.

All this was the easier to do because with wise foresight she had brought the necessary articles with her on the *Victus* from England. The ship gave up chicken, jelly, and all manner of delicacies; and, on a single day, "a thousand shirts, besides other clothing." In two weeks that "dreadful den of dirt, pestilence and death" had vanished; and in its place stood a building, light and well aired throughout, where patients lay on spotless cots, ate appetizing food from clean dishes, had their baths and their medicine at regular intervals, and never for an hour lacked any attention that would help their recovery.

But after all is said of Florence Nightingale's sympathy and her science, she owed her final triumph in the Crimea to a rarer talent, that of tactful organizing and executive power. Why was she not tethered by the system and the red tape that rendered ineffectual the best efforts of the medical men? Most things needful were in store not far from the barracks hospital. But the regular physicians could not get at them. Why could she?

In the first place she had tact enough not to offend the system. The minister of war had warned her, "a number of sentimental enthusiastic ladies turned loose into the hospital at Scutari would probably after a few days be '*mises à la porte*' by those whose business they would interrupt and whose authority they would dispute." Florence Nightingale did not at first interrupt or dispute anybody. She began by doing the neglected minor things, the things that no one else had time for. She opened windows. She scrubbed floors and walls. She laundered shirts. She peeled potatoes and boiled soup. She bathed the patients, dosed them with medicine while the worn-out surgeons were asleep, read to them, and wrote letters for them. In these activities she asked not even supplies from the system, but procured them from her own ship.

The hidebound officials were even then slow to concur. Perhaps they were jealous to see their own incompetence exposed. And there was one case,—just one—where she came to blows with them. The hospital inmates were in desperate want, and the articles for their relief were nearby in a warehouse, but the stores could not be disturbed until after inspection. Miss Nightingale tried to hasten the inspection. Failing of that, she tried to get them distributed without inspection. That also failed. "My soldiers are dying," she said. "I must have those stores." Whereupon, she called two soldiers, marched them to the warehouse, and bade them burst open the doors!

That was the kind of firm hand she could use. More often, though, she attained her ends in a peaceful way. Only a little feminine tact was necessary to bring together the dilatory members of a board and get them to unlock a storehouse. She was soon able to lay her hands on an abundance of anything the situation demanded. Then, besides her own small band of nurses, a large number of orderlies and common soldiers were, after a time, detailed to work under her direction. "Never," she says, "came from them one word or one look which a gentleman would not have used;" and many of them became attached to her with an almost slavish affection. More than that, she was, for the English at home, the one commanding figure, and her hospital office, the head-quarters of the Crimean campaign. *The Times* collected a big fund and placed it at her disposal. And all over England women were making clothing—shiploads of it—which they addressed to the soldiers in her care. "The English Nobility must have emptied their wardrobes and linen stores," said a nurse, "to send out bandages for the wounded. There was the most beautiful underclothing and the finest cambric sheets, with merely a scissors run here and there through them to insure their being used for no other purpose, some from the Queen's palace, with the royal monogram beautifully worked."

In a word, Florence Nightingale became, through her wonderful executive talent, the trusted agent of the whole British people, as powerful in the work of nursing as the commander-in-chief of the army was in fighting. Some one called her the lady-in-chief. There is perhaps not a better designation.

And the result of her efforts justified this faith. When she arrived the death rate was sixty per cent. She reduced it in a few weeks to one per cent. Nine of her nurses died on duty; other were invalided home; she herself was long fever sick and near to death. But for two years she battled against disease, always in a winning fight. She conquered disease. And it is not too much to say that she conquered the Russian army, and saved the war for the allies. No wonder England welcomed her home as one of the greatest heroines in all her history.

In 1951 Mrs. Woodham-Smith set out to present the first complete picture of Florence Nightingale. While duly praising Sir Edward Cook she noted that "there was a large body of material which, for family and personal reasons, was either not available to him or he was asked not to use." The result, a book entitled *Florence Nightingale 1820-1910*, was awarded the James Tait Black memorial Prize and has been hailed by most critics as the definitive biography, "informative, sympathetic, yet scrupulously fair and gracefully written" (Twentieth Century Authors). Mrs. Woodham-Smith, a respected authority on the role of Great Britain in the Crimean War (also wrote *The Reason Why*) and a biographer of the first order, said in 1954 that the "historian's task is to make the past live again." This she certainly accomplished. The excerpt from Chapter 10 demonstrates how Miss Nightingale's years in the Crimea were far more difficult than depicted in the previous selection. During a second period in 1855-56, for example, "she was victimized by petty jealousies, treacheries and mis-representations . . . she was miserably depressed [and] at the end of it she was obsessed by a sense of failure." But if she was disliked and distrusted by Crimean authorities, she had earned universal admiration and affection back home.

MRS. CECIL WOODHAM-SMITH

Florence Nightingale in the Crimea: National Heroine

Miss Nightingale's mission falls into two periods. There is first the period of frightful emergency during the winter of 1854-55. In Sidney Godolphin Osborne's opinion, if at that time Miss Nightingale had not been present, the hospitals must have collapsed. Every consideration but that of averting utter catastrophe went by the board, opposition died away, and she became supreme.

But as soon as things had slightly improved, official jealousy re-awoke. In the second period, from the spring of 1855 until her return to England in the summer of 1856, gratitude—except the gratitude of the troops—and admiration disappeared, and she was victimized by petty jealousies, treacheries, and misrepresentations. Throughout this second period she was miserably depressed. At the end of it she was obsessed by a sense of failure.

By the spring of 1855 she was physically exhausted. She was a slight woman who had never been robust, who was accustomed to luxury, and was now living in almost unendurable hardship. When it rained, water poured through the roof of her quarters and dripped through the floor on an officer beneath, who complained that "Miss Nightingale was pouring water on his head." The food was uneatable; the allowance of water was still one pint a head a day; the building was vermin-infested, the atmosphere in the hospital so foul that to visit the wards produced diarrhea. She never went out except to hurry over the quarter of a mile of refuse-strewn mud which separated the Barrack from the General Hospital.

When a flood of sick came in, she was on her feet for twenty-four hours at a stretch. She was known to pass eight hours on her knees dressing wounds. "She had an utter disregard of contagion," wrote Sidney Godolphin Osborne. ". . . The more awful to every sense any particular case, especially if it was that of a dying man, the more certainly might her slight form be seen bending over him, administering to his ease by every means in her power and seldom quitting his side until death released him." It was her rule never to let any man who came under her observation die alone. If he was conscious, she herself stayed beside him; if he were unconscious she sometimes allowed Mrs. Bracebridge to take her place. She estimated that during that winter she witnessed 2000 deathbeds. The worst cases she nursed herself. "I believe," wrote Dr. Pincoffs, a civilian doctor who worked in the Barrack Hospital, "that there was never a severe case of any kind that escaped her notice." One of the nurses described accompanying her on her night rounds. "It seemed an endless walk. . . . As we slowly passed along the silence was profound; very seldom did a moan or cry from those deeply suffering fall on our ears. A dim light burned here and there, Miss Nightingale carried her lantern which she would set down before she bent over any of the patients. I much admired her manner to the men—it was so tender and kind."

Her influence was extraordinary. She could make the men stop drinking, write home to their wives, submit to pain. "She was wonderful," said a veteran, "at cheering up anyone who was a bit low." The surgeons were amazed at her ability to strengthen men doomed to an operation. "The magic of her power over men was felt," writes Kinglake, "in the room—the dreaded, the bloodstained room—where operations took place. There perhaps the maimed soldier if not yet resigned to his fate, might be craving death rather than meet the knife of the surgeon, but when such a one looked and saw that the honoured Lady in Chief was patiently standing beside him—and with lips closely set and hands folded—decreeing herself to go through the pain of witnessing pain, he used to fall into the mood of obeying her silent command and—finding strange support in her presence—bring himself to submit and endure."

The troops worshiped her. "What a comfort it was to see her pass even," wrote a soldier. "She would speak to one, and nod and smile to as many more; but she could not do it all you know. We lay there by hundreds; but we could kiss her shadow as it fell and lay our heads on the pillow again content."

For her sake the troops gave up the bad language which has always been the privilege of the British private soldier. "Before she came," ran another letter, "there was cussing and swearing but after that it was as holy as a church."

When the war was over Miss Nightingale wrote: ". . . The tears come into my eyes as I think how, amidst scenes of loathsome disease and death, there rose above it all the innate dignity, gentleness and chivalry of the men (for never surely was chivalry so strikingly exemplified) shining in the midst of what must be considered the lowest sinks of human misery, and preventing instinctively the use of one expression which could distress a gentlewoman."

It was work hard enough to have crushed any ordinary woman; yet, she wrote, it was the least of her functions. The crushing burden was the administrative work. Her quarters were called the Tower of Babel. All day long a stream of callers thronged her stairs, captains of sick transports, officers of Royal Engineers, nurses, merchants, doctors, chaplains, asking for everything from writing-paper to advice on a sick man's diet, demanding shirts, splints, bandages, port wine, stoves, and butter.

She slept in the storeroom in a bed behind a screen; in the daytime she saw callers sitting and writing at a little unpainted deal table in front of it. She wore a black woollen dress, white linen collar and cuffs and apron, and a white cap under a black silk handkerchief. Every time there was a pause she snatched her pen and went on writing.

No one in the party was capable of acting as her secretary. The requisitions, the orders, the records, the immense correspondence entailed by the acknowledgement and recording of the "Free Gifts" (the voluntary contributions sent out from home), the reports, the letters, must all be written by herself. Mrs. Bracebridge had superintendence of the "Free Gift Store"; otherwise she had no assistance of any kind.

It was terribly cold, and she hated cold. There was no satisfactory stove in her quarters—one had been sent out from England, but it would not draw and she used it as a table and it was piled with papers. Her breath congealed on the air; the ink froze in the well; rats scampered in the walls and peered out from the wainscoting. Hour after hour she wrote on; the staff of the hospital declared that the light in her room was never put out. She wrote for the men, described their last hours and sent home their dying messages; she told wives of their husband's continued affection, and mothers that their sons had died holding her hand. She wrote for the nurses, many of whom had left children behind. She wrote her enormous letters to Sidney Herbert; she wrote official reports, official letters; she kept lists, filled in innumerable requisitions. Papers were piled round her in heaps; they lay on the floor, on her bed, on the chairs. Often in the morning Mrs. Bracebridge found her still in her clothes on her bed, where she had flung herself down in a stupor of fatigue.

She spared herself nothing—but the joy had gone out of the work. The high spirit, the faith which had sustained her through the first months faded as she learned the power of official intrigue.

"Alas among all the men here," she wrote to Sidney Herbert in February, 1855, "is there one really anxious for the good of these hospitals? One who is not an insincere animal at the bottom, who is not thinking of going in with the winning side whichever that is? I do believe that of all those who have been concerned in the fate of these miserable sick you and I are the only ones who really cared for them." A month later she wrote: "A great deal has been said of our self sacrifice, heroism and so forth. The real humiliation, the real hardship of this place, dear Mr. Herbert, is that we have to do with men who are neither gentlemen nor men of education nor even men of business, nor men of feeling, whose only object is to keep themselves out of blame."

She had crossed the path of such a man, and the great conflict of her mission was about to begin.

Dr. John Hall, Chief of Medical Staff of the British Expeditionary Army, had been kept occupied in the Crimea, but the hospitals of Scutari were under his control and he had no intention of allowing them to get out of hand. His name had been associated with an unsavory case in which a private stationed at Hounslow Barracks had died after receiving a flogging of 150 lashes, and he was known throughout the army as a strict disciplinarian averse to pampering the troops. He did not believe in chloroform, and in his letter of instructions to his officers at the opening of the campaign on August 3 he warned them against its use. "The smart use of the knife is a powerful stimulant and it is much better to hear a man bawl lustily than to see him sink silently into the grave." He was revengeful, powerful, a master of the confidential report. Miss Nightingale wrote to Lady Cranworth that a doctor's promotion depended "upon a trick, a caprice of the Inspector General (i.e. Dr. Hall) . . . and may be lost for an offensive word reported perhaps by an

orderly and of which he never hears and which he may never have said."
In May, 1856 she wrote: "In the last two months at this hospital alone,
two medical officers have been superseded upon evidence collected in
the above manner."

Dr. Hall entered upon his duties in the Crimea with a sense of in-
justice. He had been in Bombay, he had been due for promotion, and
he thought he deserved a post at home. He had solicited such a post
and heard with disgust that he had been appointed Chief of Medical
Staff of the British Expeditionary Army. In October, 1854, he was
sent by Lord Raglan to inspect the hospitals at Scutari. The hospitals
were then filthy and destitute. However, Dr. Hall wrote on October 20
to Dr. Andrew Smith stating he had "much satisfaction in being able to
inform him that the whole hospital establishment here (i.e. at Scutari),
has now been put on a very creditable footing and that nothing is
lacking."

It was a fatal statement. He had committed himself. Henceforward
he had to stand by what he had said, and his subordinates had to back
him up. Dr. Menzies dared not contradict Dr. Hall's specific statement.
He repeated it parrot-like to Lord Stratford, to Dr. Andrew Smith. It
was not until Sidney Herbert received Miss Nightingale's first report
that the truth was known. In December, 1854 he told Lord Raglan: "I
cannot help feeling that Dr. Hall resents offers of assistance as being
slurs on his preparations."

In the spring of 1855 Dr. Hall was boiling with rage. The Hospitals
Commission had reported unfavorably on his hospitals and, worse, he
had been censured by Lord Raglan.

The most notorious of the sick transport scandals was the case of
the *Avon*. The first man had been put on board the *Avon* at Balaclava
on November 19, 1854, the last man on December 3. The men were
laid on the bare deck without any covering but greatcoat or blanket.
One young assistant surgeon was instructed to attend to several hundred
men, and so they were left for a fortnight. The state of the ship and the
condition of the men was then indescribable. A regimental officer was
induced to visit the ship and, horrified by what he saw, galloped at once
to Lord Raglan. Though it was midnight Lord Raglan sent at once to
Dr. Hall demanding immediate action. An inquiry was held, Dr. Lawson,
the Principal Medical Officer at Balaclava, was held responsible and
severely censured for "apathy and lack of interest in he welfare of the
sick," and Dr. Hall was recommended to relieve him of his duties. Further,
in a General Order of December 13, 1854, Lord Raglan stated he could
not acquit Dr. Hall himself of blame in this matter. Dr. Hall judged the

time had come to assert himself. He was by no means beaten. He knew his powers, he had his friends, and within his own department he was invincible. Dr. Menzies the Senior Medical Officer at the Barrack Hospital had been succeeded by Dr. Forrest. After a few weeks Dr. Forrest resigned and went home in despair, and Dr. Hall then appointed Dr. Lawson to take his place. The man responsible for the *Avon* was to be Senior Medical Officer at the Barrack Hospital.

Miss Nightingale received the news with horror. "Before destroying our work Dr. Hall begins to caress us with his paws," she wrote, and she warned Sidney Herbert: "The people here will try the strength of the old system against Government reforms with a strength of purpose and a cohesion of individuals which you are not likely to give them credit for."

Dr. Lawson was a walking reminder of what the medical department could do. He had been censured and was to be relieved of his duties; he had been relieved of his duties—to assume them in a different place. Dr. Hall knew how to protect his own, and he knew how to punish the disloyal. Dr. Smith and Dr. Hall were absolute masters of the Army Medical Department, and no Nightingale power, no Sidney Herbert could save those unhappy slaves who offended their masters.

A wave of terror swept over the medical staff at Scutari. Dr. Cumming continued to call on Miss Nightingale every day, but he became nervous. He had been a member of the Hospitals Commission, but presently he was refusing to carry out his own recommendations. For example, the Hospitals Commission had stressed the urgent necessity of equiping the wards with bedding and utensils, and in March, 1855 a large quantity of hospital stores arrived with which Dr. McGrigor had the wards equipped. Dr. Cumming ordered the new equipment to be removed.

Another broken reed was Lord William Paulet, who frankly detested his job. He had been sent out because he had wealth, position, and prestige, and Major Sillery had failed because he had none of these. "Lord Wm. Paulet is appalled at the view of evils he has no idea what to do with," wrote Miss Nightingale; ". . . and then he shuts his eyes and hopes when he opens them he shall see something else." As things became more difficult, he withdrew—he put his head, she said, under his wing, spending his time with Lady Stratford picnicking along the picturesque shores of the Bosphorus, accompanied by hampers of the delicacies for which the Embassy chef was famous, ostensibly for the purpose of inspecting possible sites for convalescent hospitals. Nothing was to be expected from Lord William Paulet.

Dr. McGrigor began to succumb to Lawson's influence. He avoided Miss Nightingale; he ceased to be urgent in pressing the fulfillment of the recommendations of the Hospitals Commission. He was, she wrote, "the one of all others who really wished to help—but he was weak." She felt betrayed, though she still had her triumphs. A whole corridor which the Purveyor had delcared himself before witnesses unable to equip was fitted out by her and Mr. Macdonald from Constantinople by nightfall. "What I have done I shall continue doing," she wrote, ". . . but I am weary of this hopeless work."

Within the hospital the work of the Sanitary Commission was having rapid effect. The fearful mortality rate of February had fallen in the three weeks ending April 7 to 14½ per cent, by April 28 to 10.7 per cent, and by May 19 to 5.2 per cent.

Thanks to Miss Nightingale's purveying—the Purveyor's stores were still empty, and the authorities were slipping back into a state of mind when equipment was thought an unnecessary extravagance for a hospital—there were plenty of drugs, surgical instruments, baths, hot-water bottles, and medical comforts. Dr. Pincoffs noted that these were present in satisfactory quantities when he joined the hospital in the spring. There were also operating tables, supplied by her for the second time: the first set had been burned as firewood in the great cold of January, 1854.

Food had been miraculously improved by Alexis Soyer, the famous chef of the Reform Club, who arrived in March, 1855 with full authority from Lord Panmure. Soyer came out at his own expense attended by a "gentleman of color" as his secretary. In manner and appearance he was a comic opera Frenchman, but Miss Nightingale recognized his genius and became his friend. "Others, she wrote, "have studied cookery for the purpose of gormandizing, some for show. But none but he for the purpose of cooking large quantities of food in the most nutritive and economical manner for great quantities of people." Though the authorities received him "very coolly," Soyer was armed with authority and he proceeded to attack the kitchens of the Barrack Hospital. He composed recipes for using the army rations to make excellent soup and stews. He put an end to the frightful system of boiling. He insisted on having permanently allocated to the kitchens soldiers who could be trained as cooks. He invented ovens to bake bread and biscuits and a Scutari teapot which made and kept tea hot for fifty men. As he walked the wards with his tureens of soup, the men cheered him with three times three. Finally, he gave a luncheon attended by Lord and Lady Stratford and their suite, at which he served delicious dishes made from army rations.

In one thing Soyer failed. Like Miss Nightingale, he strongly objected to the way the meat was divided; since weight was the only criterion one man might get all bone; why should not the meat be boned, and each man receive a boneless portion, with the bones being used for broth? The answer from Dr. Cumming was that it would need a new Regulation of the Service to bone the meat.

In May, 1855 Miss Nightingale wrote to Sidney Herbert to describe "the first really satisfactory reception of sick." Two hundred men from the *Severn* transport were received, bathed, and their hair cut and cleansed. Their filthy clothes and blankets were taken from them, they were given clean hospital gowns, put into decent beds and given well-cooked nourishing food. In spite of obstacles, disappointments, opposition, she had, to this degree, succeeded.

And now that the Barrack Hospital was reasonably satisfactory, she determined to go the Crimea. There were two large hospitals at Balaclava. One, the General Hospital, had been established at the time of the British occupation in September, 1854 and, like the General Hospital at Scutari, had been intended to be the only hospital. This was the hospital in Dr. John Hall's personal charge on which the Hospitals Commission had reported adversely. The enormous numbers of sick had necessitated further accommodation, and a hospital of huts called the Castle Hospital had been erected on the heights above Balaclava harbor. Both had a staff of female nurses, and disquieting news had reached Miss Nightingale of the nurses' conduct, particularly at the General Hospital.

And now the fatal flaw in her instructions appeared, and her authority in the Crimea proved to be by no means established. Precise information as to her standing, her instructions, and the assistance to be afforded to her had been sent to Lord Raglan, Lord Stratford, and Dr. John Hall. But Lord Raglan was occupied with the problems of a disastrous campaign; Lord Stratford was indifferent; Dr. John Hall was malicious. He asserted that, as her instructions named her "Superintendent of the Female Nursing Establishment in the English Military General Hospitals in *Turkey*," she had no jurisdiction over the Crimea.

The seriousness of the situation was not appreciated at home. Mr. Augustus Stafford wrote: "The nature of her difficulties is NOT understood and perhaps never will be." Supported by Dr. Hall, nurses in the Crimea were defying her authority. One of them, Miss Clough, a "lady" of Miss Stanley's party, had broken away and gone to join Sir Colin Campbell's Hospital above Balaclava, inspired by romantic enthusiasm for the Highland Brigade. "She must be a funny fellow, she of the Highland Heights," commented Miss Nightingale. A constant rebel was

Mrs. Elizabeth Davis, the Welshwoman brought out by Mary Stanley. She had begun to dislike Miss Nightingale before she saw her. "I did not like the name of Nightingale. When I first hear a name I am very apt to know by my feelings whether I shall like the person who bears it," she wrote. She had had experience in nursing and was selected for the Barrack Hospital. Once there she proved a storm center. She refused to obey orders or to conform to the system for the distribution of the "Free Gifts." She accused Miss Nightingale of using these for her own comfort and alleged that, while the nurses were fed on filaments of the meat which had been stewed down for the patients' soup, Miss Nightingale had a French cook and three courses served up every day. Finally, she joined the party of eleven volunteers who went, against Miss Nightingale's wishes, to Balaclava in January, 1855.

Once there she made an alliance with Dr. John Hall, and another important personage in the Crimea, Mr. David Fitz-Gerald, the Purveyor-in-Chief, Mr. FitzGerald was as angrily opposed to Miss Nightingale as was Dr. Hall, and as equally determined to keep her out of the Crimea.

Elizabeth Davis, an excellent cook, had assumed command of the kitchen in Balaclava General Hospital, which she conducted with rollicking extravagance, rejoicing in feeding up the handsome young officers who were her special pets. It was Miss Nightingale's rule that none of her nurses should attend on or cook for officers except by special arrangement. At one issue Mrs. Davis received "6 dozen port wine, 6 dozen sherry, 6 dozen brandy, a cask of rice, a cask of arrowroot, a cask of sago and a box of sugar"; and her requisitions for the General Hospital were filled at once by Mr. FitzGerald without being countersigned by Dr. Hall. The situation became too much for the Superintendent, the Superior of the Sellonites, who, Miss Nightingale said, "lost her head and her health," collapsed, and went home. In her place another of Mary Stanley's party was appointed, Miss Weare, a fussy, gentle old spinster who swiftly became dominated by Mrs. Davis and Dr. Hall. Miss Weare confided to Dr. Hall how much more *natural* she found it to obey a gentleman. Miss Nightingale was very wonderful, of course, but she could not get used to taking orders from a lady.

With the "Free Gifts" Mrs. Davis and her allies were even more open-handed. In an orgy of distribution ninety bales and boxes were given away without any record of who had received them.

The "Free Gifts"—"these frightful contributions," Miss Nightingale called them, together with the labor of acknowledging them, storing them in safety, and distributing them satisfactorily, were becoming the bane of her life. Ever since November, 1854, parcels had been sent from England for the troops. "There is not a small town, not a parish in England from which we have not received contributions," she wrote in May, 1855, "not one of these is worth its freight, but the smaller the value, of course, the greater the importance the contributors attach to it. If you knew the trouble of landing, of unpacking, of acknowledging! The good that has been done here has been done by money, money purchasing articles in Constantinople.

Among the "Free Gifts" were articles of value. Queen Victoria had sent a number of water-beds; there were also provisions, groceries, wine, brandy, soup, and clothing. To keep a check was difficult; the store, like every other place in Scutari, was overrun by rats, and the Maltese, Greek, and Turkish laborers who worked round the hospital were dishonest almost without exception. After her arrival on November 5, 1854, Miss Nightingale kept an exact record of every article received and issued by her. After February 15, 1855 Mrs. Bracebridge was left in sole charge.

On May 2, 1855, she sailed from Scutari for Balaclava in the *Robert Lowe.* "Poor old Flo," she wrote to her mother, "steaming up the Bosphorus and across the Black Sea with four nurses, two cooks, and a boy to Crim Tartary . . . in the Robert Lowe or Robert Slow (for an exceedingly slow boat she is), . . . taking back 420 of her patients, a draught of convalescents returning to their regiments to be shot at again. 'A Mother in Israel,' Pastor Fliedner called me; a Mother in the Coldstreams, is the more appropriate appellation."

Besides Soyer and a French chef, the party included Soyer's secretary, the "gentleman of color," Mr. Bracebridge and a boy named Robert Robinson, an invalided drummer from the 68th Light Infantry. He described himself as Miss Nightingale's "man"—Soyer could not resist asking him whether he was twelve years old yet—and was accustomed to explain that he had "forsaken his instruments in order to devote his civil and military career to Miss Nightingale." He carried her letters and messages, escorted her when she went from the Barrack Hospital to the General Hospital, and had charge of the lamp which she carried at night. Among the Nightingale papers is a manuscript account of his experiences during the campaign, entitled "Robert Robinson's Memoir." He was, said Soyer, "a regular *enfant de troupe,* full of wit and glee."

On May 5, six months after her arrival at Constantinople—"and what the disappointments of those six months have been no one could tell," she wrote, "but still I am not dead but alive"—the *Robert Lowe* anchored in Balaclava harbor. Balaclava was crammed to overflowing, and she was invited by the Captain to make her quarters on board the ship, which soon, wrote Soyer, resembled a floating drawing-room, as doctors, senior officers, and officials, including Sir John McNeill of the Tulloch and McNeill Commission and Dr. Sutherland of the Sanitary Commission, came to pay their respects. In the afternoon, escorted by a number of gentlemen, she went ashore to report herself to Lord Raglan. She appeared, says Soyer, in a "genteel Amazone," and rode a "very pretty mare which by its gambols and caracoling seemed proud to carry its noble charge." Lord Raglan being away for the day, she decided to visit the mortar battery outside Sebastopol. The astonishing sight of a lady in Balaclava accompanied by a crowd of gentlemen, many of them in glittering uniforms, produced "an extraordinary effect." The news spread like wildfire that the lady was Miss Nightingale, and the soldiers rushed from their tents and "cheered her to the echo with three times three." At the Mortar Battery Soyer requested her to ascend the rampart and seat herself on the center mortar, "to which she very gracefully acceded." He then "boldly exclaimed, 'Gentlemen, behold this amiable lady sitting fearlessly upon the terrible instrument of war! Behold the heroic daughter of England, the soldiers' friend!'" Three cheers were given by all. Meanwhile five or six of her escort had picked bouquets of the wild lilies and orchids which carpeted the plateau. She was requested to choose the one she liked best and responded by gathering them all in her arms.

The party then cantered home, Miss Nightingale looking strangely exhausted. It was, she said, the unaccustomed fresh air.

The next morning, accompanied by Soyer, she began her inspection. It was a depressing task. The hospitals were dirty and extravagantly run, the nurses inefficient and undisciplined. She was received with hostility and, at the General Hospital, with insolence. "I should have as soon expected to see the Queen here as you," said Mrs. Davis.

She ignored hostility and rudeness. She got out plans with Soyer's assistance for new extra diet kitchens at the General Hospital. She decided Miss Weare must be replaced—the General Hospital was evidently out of hand. She then went up to the Castle Hospital, the new hospital of huts where Mrs. Shaw Stewart (the "Mrs." was a courtesy title), a difficult woman herself, was having a difficult time. Mrs. Shaw Stewart, one of Mary Stanley's party, was one of the few women of social position who had any real experience in nursing. She was the sister of Sir Michael Shaw Stewart, M.P., and had undergone training in Germany and nursed in a London hospital. She was skillful, kind, a magnificent worker, but she would be a martyr. Do what her friends would, conciliate her, defer to her, coax her, she maintained she was being ill-treated. At the Castle Hospital she had no need to imagine persecution, for Dr. Hall was making her work as difficult as possible. He caused immense inconvenience by insisting that all her requisitions must be sent to him personally. Work which the Sanitary Commission had directed was not even started, her kitchens were inadequate, the Purveyor habitually held up her supplies, and finally, Dr. Hall made a practice of sending her messages of criticism through her staff.

Miss Nightingale gathered herself together to do battle, but before anything could be accomplished she collapsed. After seeing Mrs. Shaw Stewart, she had admitted great weakness and fatigue, and the next day, while interviewing Miss Weare, she fainted. The Senior Medical Officer from the Balaclava General Hospital was hastily summoned; after he had called two other doctors into consultation, a statement was issued that Miss Nightingale was suffering from Crimean fever.

All Balaclava, says Soyer, was in an uproar. It was decided that she must be removed from the ship. The harbor was being cleansed by the Sanitary Commission, and the men working to remove the ghastly debris found the stench so horrible that they constantly fainted and had to receive an official issue of brandy. She must be taken to the pure air of the Castle Hospital on the heights. A solemn cortège transported her from the ship, four soldiers carrying her on a stretcher and Dr. Anderson and Mrs. Roberts walking by her side; Soyer's secretary— Soyer himself was away—held an umbrella over her head, and Robert Robinson walked behind in tears, being, in his own words, "not strong enough to help carry or tall enough to hold the umbrella." By this time she was delirious and very ill. At Balaclava the troops seemed in mourning, and at Scutari the men when they heard the news, "turned their faces to the wall and cried. All their trust was in her," a Sergeant wrote home.

For more than two weeks, nursed by Mrs. Roberts, she hovered between life and death. In her delirium she was constantly writing. It was found impossible to keep her quiet unless she wrote, so she was given pen and paper; among the Nightingale papers are sheets covered with feverish notes. She thought her room was full of people demanding supplies, that an engine was inside her head, that a Persian adventurer came and stood beside her bed and told her that Mr. Bracebridge had given him a draft for 300,000 pounds sterling, and she wrote to Sir John McNeill asking him to deal with the man because he had been in Persia. In the height of the fever all her hair was cut off. The news

went round the camp, and Colonel Sterling wrote that he heard the
Bird had had to have her head shaved—would she wear a wig or a
helmet!

At home the tidings were received with consternation, and when
it was known that she was recovering strangers passed on the good
news to each other in the streets.

On May 24 a horseman wrapped in a cloak rode up to her hut
and knocked. Mrs. Roberts sprang out—"Hist, hist, don't make such
a horrible noise as that, my man." He asked if this were Miss Nightingale's hut. Mrs. Roberts said it was, and he tried to walk in. Mrs. Roberts
pushed him back. "And pray who are you?" she asked. "Oh, only a
soldier, but I must see her, I have come a long way, my name is Raglan,
she knows me very well." "Oh, Mrs. Roberts it is Lord Raglan," called
Miss Nightingale. He came in and, drawing up a stool to her bedside,
talked to her at length. That night he telegraphed home that Miss
Nightingale was out of danger, and on May 28 Queen Victoria was
"truly thankful to learn that that excellent and valuable person Miss
Nightingale is safe."

She was frantic to settle the urgent problems at Balaclava, but her
weakness was so extreme that she could not feed herself or raise her
voice above a whisper. The doctors advised her to go to England, or
failing that to Switzerland. She refused, and Mrs. Bracebridge, who
had hastened from Scutari to look after her, pointed out that she
was such an execrable sailor that a long sea voyage in her present
state might well kill her. It was arranged that she should be taken to
Scutari on a transport and occupy a house belonging to Mr. Sabin,
who had gone home on sick leave.

A curious incident followed. Dr. Hadley, the Senior Medical
Officer at the Castle Hospital, had attended her. Dr. Hadley was a
friend of Dr. John Hall, and the two doctors selected the transport,
the *Jura*, on which she was to go to Scutari. She was actually on board
when Mr. Bracebridge discovered that the *Jura* was not calling at
Scutari but going direct to England. Miss Nightingale was hurried off
the transport in a fainting condition by Mr. Bracebridge and Lord
Ward, and crossed to Scutari on Lord Ward's steam yacht. On October 19, 1855, she wrote to Sidney Herbert: "It was quite true that
Doctors Hall and Hadley sent for a list of vessels going home, and
chose one, the Jura, which was not going to stop at Scutari *because* it
was not going to stop at Scutari, and put me on board her for England."

The voyage was rough, the yacht was kept at sea an extra day,
and Miss Nightingale was dreadfully ill. At Scutari her weakness and

exhaustion were such that she was unable to speak. She was terribly changed, emaciated, white-faced under the handkerchief tied closely round her head to conceal her shorn hair. Two relays of guardsmen carried her to Mr. Sabin's house on a stretcher. Twelve private soldiers divided the honor of carrying her baggage. The stretcher was followed by a large number of men, absolutely silent and many openly in tears. "I do not remember anything so gratifying to the feelings," wrote Soyer, "as that simple though grand procession."

Mr. Sabin's house had windows opening on to the Bosphorus—the most famous view in the world which, she said, she had never had time to look at—and a green tree in a garden behind. Here she began slowly to recover.

For the next few weeks she lived in the world of the convalescent, a world filled with small things. Sidney Herbert had sent her a terrier from England, and she had an owl, given her by the troops to take the place of Athena, and a baby. The baby belonged to a Sergeant Brownlow, and while its mother was washing for the hospital used to spend its day in a sort of Turkish wooden pen which she could see from her bed. Its merits, she wrote afterwards, were commemorated in the chapter on "Minding Baby" in *Notes on Nursing*. Parthe composed and illustrated and sent her "The Life and Death of Athena, an Owlet." Mrs. Bracebridge read it aloud while Miss Nightingale alternately laughed and cried and noticed how the terrier kept fidgeting about and drawing attention to himself, "knowing by instinct we were reading about something we loved very much and being jealous." By July she was better and had decided she was not going away anywhere. "If I go, all this will go to pieces," she wrote to Parthe on July 9. Dr. Sutherland told her the fever had saved her life by forcing her to rest and implored her to spare herself. She dared not. She had been compelled to leave the Crimea before she had settled anything, and she was receiving reports that the situation was going from bad to worse. Every day her authority was being more flagrantly disregarded. As soon as was humanly possible, she must go back to Balaclava and fight it out.

She spent a few days at Therapia with Mrs. Bracebridge, then returned to Mr. Sabin's house and resumed ordinary life. She contrived to give an impression of complete recovery. Lothian Nicholson visited her on his way up to the Crimea and was "quite enthusiastic about her good looks." Her cropped hair was growing in little curls which gave her a curiously touching and childish appearance.

But as she recovered the stormclouds gathered. She was about to enter the most difficult and exhausting phase of her mission. During her illness Lord Raglan died and was succeeded by General Simpson, a soldier of many years seniority who had barely seen active service.

General Simpson's intelligence was not great, his social position inferior; he was against new-fangled notions of pampering the troops, and Miss Nightingale never succeeded in establishing the personal contact she had enjoyed with Lord Raglan. "The man who was Lord FitzRoy Somerset" (Lord Raglan as youngest son of the Duke of Beaufort bore the title of Lord FitzRoy Somerset before being created Baron Raglan in 1852) "would naturally not be above interesting himself in hospital matters and a parcel of women—while the man who was James Simpson would essentially think it infra dig," she wrote in November, 1855. Moreover, for some reason the official instructions as to her position and authority which had been sent by Sidney Herbert when Secretary at War to Lord Raglan were not passed on to General Simpson.

She learned that in the Crimea the kitchens which she had planned with Soyer had not been built, supplies were still being withheld from Mrs. Shaw Stewart, the conduct of the nurses was still unsatisfactory. In July she sent up a French man-cook, to whom she paid 100 pounds sterling a year out of her own private income, but the authorities refused to employ him. She requested that the ineffectual Miss Weare should be relieved as Superintendent of the General Hospital. Dr. Hall's reply was to appoint Miss Weare Superintendent of the Monastery Hospital, a new hospital for ophthalmic cases and convalescents, and ignore her request.

As she was bracing herself to gather strength and return to the Crimea, a fresh blow fell. The Bracebridges wished to go home. For nine months they had shared the fearful sights, the horrible smells, the uneatable food, the insolence, the petty slights, and the perpetual rudeness. They had endured, toiled, sacrificed themselves, and yet—they had not been a complete success. Their devotion was as strong as ever, Miss Nightingale's affection as grateful. "No one can tell what she has been to me," she wrote of Selina, but Selina had muddled the "Free Gift" store, and Mr. Bracebridge's relations with the officials were increasingly unhappy.

Though she was barely convalescent, she would not hear of delay in the Bracebridges' departure. Everything was made easy. It was given out that they were going home for a few months and would come back in the autumn, but she knew they would never return. As soon as they sailed on July 28 she went back to her quarters at the Barrack Hospital, retaining Mr. Sabin's house and sending her nurses there by turns to have a rest.

The medical authorities did not welcome her. They felt that the state of the hospital was now satisfactory and her help was not needed; there was an unwillingness to consult her and an outbreak of complaints. Orderlies caught in wrongdoing had only to say Miss Nightingale had given the order to be exonerated. Some of the admirable work of the Sanitary Commission was being undone. The engineering works were not completed, and the men began once more to drink water that looked like barley water. Trouble in controlling the nurses was continuous. Two nurses broke out one Saturday night and were brought back dead drunk. "A great disappointment to me," wrote Miss Nightingale, "as they were both good natured hard working women."

Nurses who did not drink got married. Lady Alicia Blackwood related that one morning six of Miss Nightingale's best nurses came into her room followed by six corporals or sergeants to announce their impending weddings. On one occasion an emissary from a Turkish official called on Miss Nightingale with an offer to purchase a particularly plump nurse for his master's harem.

She lost one of her best nurses on August 9 when Mrs. Drake, from St. John's House, died of cholera at Balaclava. Next she was involved in unpleasantness through the death of Miss Clough, who had got into difficulties on the "Highland Heights." She disliked living in a hut, could not control the orderlies, was accused of financial irregularities, quarreled with everyone, fell ill, and asked to be sent home. On the boat she became worse and was put ashore at Scutari, where she died. Miss Nightingale had to receive her body, arrange her funeral, communicate news of her death to her relations at home, and straighten her affairs.

Much more serious trouble followed. After Mrs. Bracebridge went home, Miss Nightingale appointed a Miss Salisbury to take charge of the "Free Gift" store at a salary. From the moment she took up her post, she began writing letters home accusing Miss Nightingale of neglecting the patients, of wasting the "Free Gifts," and of having been concerned in Miss Clough's sudden death. These letters found their way to Mary Stanley, who was now in London. Miss Salisbury next began thieving from the store on a considerable scale. A search was ordered not only of Miss Salisbury's room but of the room of two Maltese kitchen-workers whom she had introduced. The results were staggering. The beds of the Maltese were found to be entirely constructed of piles of stolen goods, while in Miss Salisbury's room every box, every package, every crevice and cranny was crammed.

Miss Nightingale summoned the Military Commandant. Lord William Paulet had just gone home and had been replaced by General

Storks, a man of first-rate ability and one of her staunch admirers. The wretched Miss Salisbury was now groveling on the floor, sobbing, screaming, and clutching at Miss Nightingale's feet, imploring her not to prosecute, but to send her home, now, at once, immediately. A grave mistake was made. Miss Nightingale wished above all things to avoid a scandal, and she and General Storks agreed that the wisest course was to send Miss Salisbury home with as little fuss as possible. She sailed immediately. But after she had gone, it was discovered that she had been stealing not only Free Gifts but government stores as well. General Storks suggested that in order to trace the stores and discover her accomplices her desk, which in the flurry of departure she had left behind, should be opened and searched and letters that came for her should be opened and read.

When Miss Salisbury arrived in England, she declared she had been ill-treated. The gifts were decaying in the store because Miss Nightingale refused to let them be used, or used them herself, and Miss Salisbury had abstracted them in order to give them to the poor fellows for whom they were intended. Why, she demanded, had not the police been called in if what Miss Nightingale asserted was true? Miss Salisbury was soon in conference with Mary Stanley, and a formal complaint against Miss Nightingale was drawn up and submitted to the War Office.

Within the War Office there were two parties, a reform party and an anti-reform party. Sending out four Commissions of Inquiry, or sending out even Miss Nightingale herself, had not been accomplished without battles. The anti-reform party had been defeated and were ready to use any weapon that came to hand. At their head was Mr. Benjamin Hawes, Permanent Under-Secretary at the War Office.

Miss Salisbury's complaint was submitted to Mr. Hawes, and he chose to take it very seriously. An official letter was written to Miss Nightingale and General Storks—who had schemes for the reform of army administration which Mr. Hawes did not find sympathetic—not inviting a report but requesting them to justify their conduct.

Miss Nightingale had now to add to her labors the fearful task of straightening out the "Free Gift" store. Miss Salisbury's accusations and the action of the War Office became known in London, and her family blamed the Bracebridges; W.E.N., wrote Uncle Sam, *"would give out against good B."* Someone must go out to be with Florence. Aunt Mai tactfully suggested she should go out for a short time until the Bracebridges returned—ostensibly in the autumn—and Uncle Sam rather unwillingly consented.

On September 16 Aunt Mai arrived at Scutari. She burst into

tears at her first sight of Florence, altered by her illness, thin and worn, and with her hair cut short looking curiously like the child of thirty years ago. The web of partisan intrigue, the party thwartings, irritations, and discourtesies in which she was forced to live horrified Aunt Mai. "The public generally imagine her by the soldier's bedside," she wrote on September 18, 1855; ". . . how easy, how satisfactory if that were all. The quantity of writing, the quantity of talking is the weary work, the dealing with the mean, the selfish, the incompetent."

The pressure of work was enormous. During her first week Aunt Mai recorded getting up at 6 A.M. and copying until 11 P.M., and next day getting up at 5 A.M. and copying again until 11 P.M.

At the beginning of October Miss Nightingale went back to the Crimea, where a new tempest had blown up, with, in its center, Rev. Mother Bridgeman—"Mother Brickbat." Miss Nightingale had never succeeded in persuading Mother Bridgeman to acknowledge her authority. Mother Bridgeman had gone with her nuns to Koulali, where they issued "extras," wine, invalid food, and clothing at their own discretion and without a requisition from the doctor in charge. Lord Panmure, on his appointment as Secretary of State for War, had asked Miss Nightingale to relinquish Koulali, and she had consented. But the lavishness there became such a scandal that the Principal Medical Officer insisted that the Scutari system must be adopted. The nuns then resigned, saying their usefulness was destroyed.

At the end of September, 1855, Miss Nightingale had learned that Mother Bridgeman and her nuns, without either informing her or asking her permission, had gone to the General Hospital, Balaclava, where Mother Bridgeman was to be Superintendent. She asked Dr. Hall for an explanation and he alleged that he had written her a letter asking for more nurses, but had had no reply and had been forced to take action. No such letter had been received.

Mother Bridgeman then wrote announcing that four of her nuns who were still working at the General Hospital, Scutari, were to proceed to Balaclava. Miss Nightingale pointed out that to remove nurses who were engaged in her service was against all rules. Mother Bridgeman refused to give way, and Miss Nightingale appealed to Lord Stratford; it was, she wrote, impossible for her to carry on her work if interference with the control of her nurses was permitted. At the same time, in a private letter, she told him that she was quite ready to arrange for the nuns to go to Balaclava; if any women were to be at the General Hospital, Balaclava, she thought nuns the least undesirable, but arrangements must be made through her and not over her head. Lord Stratford hastened in complimentary terms to assure her of his entire agreement, but informed her that she should approach not himself but General Storks.

When Miss Nightingale considered the situation, she came to the conclusion that her personal resentment must be swallowed. Wide implications were involved. The new recruits brought out to replace the army which had perished in the winter of 1854-55 were largely Irish and Catholics, and it was already being said that they were being deprived of spiritual ministrations. "Had we more nuns," she wrote to Mrs. Herbert in November, 1855, "it would be very desirable, to diminish disaffection. But *just not* the Irish ones. The wisest thing the War Office could do now would be to send out a few more of the Bermondsey nuns to join those already at Scutari and counter balance the influence of the *Irish* ones, who hate their soberer sisters with the mortal hatred, which, I believe, only Nuns and Household Servants *can* feel towards each other."

She returned to the Crimea determined, in her favorite phrase, to "arrange things." On September 8 Sebastopol had quietly and ingloriously fallen, evacuated by the enemy, and the end of the war was only a question of time. General Simpson had resigned his command and gone home suffering from Crimean diarrhea and been succeeded by Sir William Codrington. She was desperately anxious to keep things together, not to come to shipwreck at the eleventh hour. She was ready to conciliate—to conciliate Dr. Hall, conciliate Mother Bridgeman, conciliate Mr. FitzGerald, the Purveyor.

The weather was bad, sailing delayed and the passage finally made in a gale. She was prostrated. Outside Balaclava it proved impossible to make the narrow opening to the harbor or even to bring out a tug. While the transport rose and fell on huge swells, a small boat was brought alongside. A sailor held her over the side of the ship, and as the boat rose dropped her into it.

At first it seemed that she might succeed in "arranging things." It was an advantage to be without Mr. Bracebridge: "I find much less difficulty in getting on here without him that with him," she wrote in November, 1855. "A woman obtains that from military courtesy (if she does not shock either their habits of business or their caste prejudice), which a man who pitted the civilian against the military element and the female against the doctors, partly from temper, partly from policy, effectually hindered." On the surface she was on friendly terms with Dr. Hall and Mr. FitzGerald. In fact, Mr. FitzGerald went so far as to confess to her he hoped that Mother Bridgeman's nuns would not import extravagant Koulali habits into Balaclava.

And then a copy of *The Times* for October 16, 1855, arrived at Balaclava, and all her work was undone. It contained a report of a lecture given by Mr. Bracebridge at the Town Hall, Coventry. Everything Mr. Bracebridge had previously said, which she had implored him to refrain from saying, he had now repeated publicly. The lecture was a furious and inaccurate attack on the British Army authorities and the British Army doctors. The harm done was incalculable. Other papers reprinted Mr. Bracebridge's allegations, and it was believed that Miss Nightingale had instigated a Press attack on the Army Medical Department. Everything asserted of her by Dr. Hall was felt to be justified.

"When one reads such twaddling nonsense," wrote Dr. Hall to Dr. Andrew Smith, "as that uttered by Mr. Bracebridge and which was so much lauded in the 'Times' because the garrulous old gentleman talked about Miss Nightingale putting hospitals containing three or four thousand patients in order in a couple of days by means of the 'Times' fund, one cannot suppress a feeling of contempt for the man who indulges in such exaggerations and pity for the ignorant multitude who are deluded by these fairy tales."

Angry as Dr. Hall was, he was no more furious than Miss Nightingale herself. On November 5 she told Mr. Bracebridge she wished for no "mere irresponsibility of opposition." She objected in the strongest possible manner to his lecture, "*First,* because it is not our business and I have expressly denied being a medical officer . . . *secondly,* because it justifies all the attacks made against us for unwarrantable interference and criticism, and *thirdly,* because I believe it to be utterly unfair." Alas, the damage had been done, and it was irremediable. She contemplated the wreckage of her endeavors with despair.

"I have been appointed a twelvemonth today," she wrote to Aunt Mai, "and what a twelvemonth of dirt it has been, of experience which would sadden not a life but eternity. Who has ever had a sadder experience. Christ was betrayed by one, but my cause has been betrayed by everyone—ruined, destroyed, betrayed by everyone alas one may truly say excepting Mrs. Roberts, Rev. Mother and Mrs. Stewart. All the rest, Weare, Clough, Salisbury, Stanley et id genus omne where are they? And Mrs. Stewart is more than half mad. A cause which is supported by a mad woman and twenty fools must be a falling house. . . . Dr. Hall is dead against me, justly provoked but not by me. He descends to every meanness to make my position more difficult."

As if she had not enough to endure, she was taken ill again and forced to enter the Castle Hospital with severe sciatica. Minus the pain, which was great, she wrote to Mrs. Bracebridge that the attack did not seem to have damaged her much. "I have now had all that this climate can give. Crimean fever, Dysentery, Rheumatism and believe myself thoroughly acclimatised and ready to stand out the war with any man."

In a week she was up and working again, ignoring personal humiliations as long as female nursing in military hospitals might emerge as a unified undertaking at the end of the War. No official statement came to establish her authority, and Dr. Hall gave out that she was an adventuress and to be treated as such. Minor officials treated her with vulgar impertinence. The Purveyor refused to honor her drafts. When she went to the General Hospital, she was kept waiting.

But she would not be provoked. She persisted in visiting Mother Bridgeman, and when Sister Winifred, a lay sister from Mother Bridgeman's party, died of cholera she went to the funeral and joined in the prayers. "Mother Brickbat's conduct has been neither that of a Christian, a gentlewoman, or even a woman," Miss Nightingale wrote to Mrs. Herbert. "At the same time I am the best personal friends with the Revd. Brickbat and I have even offered to put up a cross to poor Winifred to which she has deigned no reply. But anything to avoid a woman's quarrel which *can* be done or submitted to on my part *shall* be done— and submitted to."

All she had accomplished by coming to the Crimea, she wrote, was that the extra diet kitchens which should have been erected in May were erected in November. At the end of November she was hastily summoned back to Scutari, where a new cholera epidemic had broken out. Before she left, she wrote to Sidney Herbert: "There is not an official who would not burn me like Joan of Arc if he could, but they know the War Office cannot turn me out because the country is with me—that is my position." The admiration and affection with which the people of England regarded her roused in the Crimean authorities dislike and distrust. But their masters at home, Ministers to whom public opinion was of importance, had a different outlook, and in November, when her prestige in the Crimea had never been so low or her difficulties so great, an astonishing demonstration of public feeling and affection in England placed her in the position of a national heroine whom no one could afford to ignore.

Philip A. Kalisch is Associate Professor of History and
Politics of Nursing at the School of Nursing, University
of Michigan, Ann Arbor and his wife Beatrice is Shirley C.
Titus Professor of Nursing and Chairperson of the Parent-
Child Nursing Department there. Co-authors of many
articles in the History of Nursing area (mostly on nursing
in wartime) they recently came out with a textbook entitled *The Advance of American Nursing* (1978). In their
opening chapter, from which this excerpt is taken, they
have effectively and succinctly summarized the impact
of Florence Nightingale on the history of American nursing.
Because of the expertise and mass of documentation
accumulated by the Kalischs on military nursing, the
assessment of Miss Nightingale's role in the Crimean War
is particularly effective. In their words:

> While the Crimean War caused untold suffering, it also led
> to one of the greatest humanitarian advances of history: mod-
> ern military nursing, from which developed professional
> nursing in general.

PHILIP and BEATRICE KALISCH

"The Birth of Modern Nursing"
Florence Nightingale: Pioneer

The Birth of Modern Nursing

During the nineteenth century deaconess orders, which had previously
existed back near the time of Christ, were revived by Protestant churches
that felt the need for the assistance of women in conducting religious
work.

The first modern order of deaconesses was established in 1836
by the German Pastor Theodor Fliedner of Kaiserwerth, who needed
an organized corps of nurses for his new infirmary. This experiment
proved so successful that it was immediately copied by Lutheran
organizations in other parts of Europe. As instituted by Pastor Fliedner,
the Order of Deaconesses of the Rhenish Province of Westphalia comprised three classes of members: the first class devoted itself to the
care of the sick poor and to the rescue of fallen women by the means
of Magdalen homes; the second class served as teachers; the third class,
known as visitation deaconesses, assumed the responsibilities of regular
parochial work.

It was in the little German town of Kaiserwerth that the modern movement for nursing education began. Here Pastor Fliedner and his devoted wife Friederike established a refuge for discharged prisoners. Aroused by the lack of facilities for the care of the sick and by physicians' bitter complaints "of the hireling service by day and night, of the drunkenness and immorality of the attendants" then available, they opened a small hospital with a training school for deaconesses in 1836. The first candidate, Gertrude Reichardt, was so disheartened when she saw the sparse facilities and poor equipment—"a shabby table, some brokenbacked chairs, worn-out knives, two-pronged forks, worm-eaten beds and appliances to match"—that she was about to return home in despair. But soon a large bundle arrived containing a quantity of new bed linen, clothing, and ward fittings. She regarded this windfall as a providential sign and remained to become the first of the deaconesses dedicated to a new ideal of nursing. Thus, the efforts of the Fliedners resulted in the birth of modern nursing and prepared the way for Florence Nightingale.

Eighteen years later, soon after the outbreak of the Crimean War—in which Britain, France, and Turkey fought against Russia for control of access to the Mediterranean from the Black Sea—ugly rumors of the neglect and mismanagement of casualties began to reach England. Reports dispatched by William Howard Russell, special correspondent to the *London Times*, and printed on October 9 and 12, 1854, revealed that the hospitals contained "neither surgeons, dressers, nurses, nor the commonest appliance of a workhouse sick ward." Later, after observing that the French were receiving nursing care from the Sisters of Charity, Russell demanded, "Why have we no Sisters of Charity?"

In regard to conditions in British hospitals, correspondent Russell wrote that "the commonest accessories of a hospital are wanting; there is not the least attention paid to decency or cleanliness; the stench is appalling; the fetid air can barely stuggle out to taint the atmosphere, save through the chinks in the walls and roofs; and, for all I can observe, these men die without the slightest effort being made to save them." He added that "the sick appear to be tended by the sick, the dying by the dying."

The corridors and wards of the Barrack Hospital at Scutari were paved with dirty broken stones. The damp, filthy building was in a bad state of repair and infested with rats and vermin. Sanitary arrangements were appalling. No steps had been taken to clean the rooms, beds, and bedding, and all necessary equipment was lacking. Russell noted that "the manner in which the sick and wounded are treated is worthy only of the savage . . . The hospitals have not the commonest appliances of a workhouse sick ward."

The Duke of Newcastle, as Secretary of War, was responsible for the administration of the Army, and Sir Sidney Herbert, as Secretary at War, was placed in charge of its finances. Even though Newcastle was grossly overworked, he quickly decided to send a commission to investigate Russell's allegations. Meanwhile Herbert, who for years had been interested in the care of the sick, took control of the situation. Russell had contrasted the deplorable medical and sanitary conditions of the British with those of the French, for whom 50 Sisters of Charity were providing admirable nursing care. Herbert saw no reason why Britain too should not send a group of women nurses. He knew that there would be some opposition in Parliament, but he was determined to make the attempt.

Florence Nightingale: Pioneer

Herbert's thoughts turned at once to Miss Florence Nightingale. On Sunday, October 15, 1854, he wrote to Miss Nightingale explaining the situation and the need for women nurses in the Crimea. He claimed that she was the only person in England capable of organizing and supervising such a plan. "Would you listen to the request to go and superintend the whole thing," he stated, "deriving your authority from the Government, your position would secure the respect and consideration of everyone." With Miss Nightingale's acceptance of this challenge, nursing took one of its longest steps forward.

Florence Nightingale had been born in Florence 34 years before, on May 13, 1820, and had been named after the city of her birth. Born of wealthy, influential English parents, she was raised in England and, unlike the average English girl of the time, received a thorough education. She and the only other child of the family, Parthenope, were tutored by governesses, and as the girls grew older, their father took an active part in their education. Early in her teenage years Florence mastered the fundamentals of Greek and Latin, read Plato, studied history, mathematics, and philosophy, and wrote essays on subjects designated by her father. She was a shy, sensitive child, inclined to be pensive and somewhat morbid.

Soon after her seventeenth birthday Florence returned to Italy. Later she took other trips with her parents or in the company of family friends. During these travels, in addition to the usual itinerary of art, architecture, and nature study, she invariably took notes on the laws and social conditions of the lands which she visited. Her sister, on the other hand, as an average girl of a prominent family, preferred social activities. Upon returning from their first continental trip, the girls were presented at Court.

At an early age, Florence expressed to her parents a desire to enter the nursing field, but they were convinced that nursing was a profession suited only for women like Sairy Gamp. While Florence fully appreciated her parents' viewpoint, she determined that it would not be necessary for her to degrade herself in order to become a nurse. Moreover, she considered it unfair to condemn an occupation because of its existing poor reputation. Rather, she thought it better to correct the evils in nursing.

Her decision to train in an English hospital at the age of 25, nine years prior to Herbert's summons, was met by the determined objections of her mother, who naturally expected Florence to marry wisely and to assume her inherited place in society. Florence rejected matrimony, however, and took advantage of every opportunity to acquaint herself with nursing conditions.

In the autumn of 1849, Miss Nightingale departed on a tour with family friends. They wintered in Egypt, and Florence spent time in Alexandria with the Sisters of Charity of Saint Vincent de Paul. Spring, 1850, found her in Athens, from where she set out, unaccompanied, for Kaiserswerth. Arriving in July, 1850, she remained there for two weeks and came away firmly resolved to return there to train as a nurse, despite the objections of her family.

The following year, when her ailing sister Parthenope was about to journey to the mineral springs of Carlsbad, Florence insisted on going to Kaiserwerth for nurses' training while Mrs. Nightingale and Parthenope stayed at the resort. Permission was granted on condition that no one outside the family was to know where she went. Florence reached the deaconess institution early in July, 1851, and stayed three months.

Finally, after Florence returned from Germany and the Nightingales were settled back home in England, provisions were made for her to enter her chosen profession. After arrangements had been made for Florence to go to France to work with several Catholic nursing sisters, her mother induced her to postpone the trip. It was 1853 before she reached Paris, where, granted an official permit, she inspected hospitals and religious institutions and observed surgeons at their work. While in France she negotiated for a position in England as superintendent of the Establishment for Gentlewomen During Illness, a charity hospital for governesses run by titled ladies. She assumed this position upon her return to London, but friends soon persuaded her to leave the institution, for she was handicapped by an intolerant board of directors with little knowledge of good hospital management. Negotiations were under way for her appointment as the superintendent of nurses at King's College Hospital when the outbreak of the Crimean War presented her with a brilliant and unexpected opportunity for achievement.

At Herbert's insistence, the British government conferred on Miss Nightingale the inspiring title "Superintendent of the Female Nursing Establishment of the English General Hospitals in Turkey." This lofty title was a misnomer, for there was not yet any female nursing establishment to superintend, but this deficiency was soon remedied by a frantic recruiting drive in London. Two days after receipt of her orders, on October 21, 1854, the newly appointed superintendent set out for the Dardanelles with 38 self-proclaimed nurses of varied experience, of whom 24 were nuns. The other 14 also claimed some nursing experience—which generally meant very little.

Florence Nightingale and her nursing force arrived at Scutari, a suburb of Constantinople on the Asiatic side of the Bosphorus, on November 4, 1854. It was here that the British military hospital had been established in a huge building called Selimah Kishler. Previously housing Turkish artillery, it had been requisitioned because it had appeared to offer suitable accommodations. Renamed the "Barrack," this building had acquired an ignominious reputation. There were no beds, no furniture, no eating utensils, no medical supplies, and no blankets. The latrines were clogged and the tubs standing in the passage were never emptied. Men lay naked on the floor in their own excrement. It was later estimated that three-quarters of all the casualties suffered by the British Army in the Crimean War resulted from such diseases as dysentery, typhoid, and cholera, which were contracted in the hospital. The Barrack Hospital had proved to be a death trap rather than a sanatorium. Moreover, it had been the subject of extremely unfavorable journalistic reports, much to the consternation of Dr. John Hall, Chief of Medical Staff for the British Expeditionary Force.

Even though some medical officers complained to each other about the ineptitude of the Medical Department and privately acknowledged both the verity of William Howard Russell's exposés in the *Times* and the value of sending Miss Nightingale and her nurses, the majority resented this outside interference and drew together into "a defensive phalanx" to justify and protect themselves. Most medical officers, like Dr. Hall, regarded Miss Nightingale as an intruder who would undermine military authority. A powerful, mutual hatred

soon developed between the two. When Dr. Hall was awarded the
K.C.B. (Knight Commander of the Order of the Bath), Miss Nightingale
sarcastically referred to him as the "Knight of the Crimean Burial
Grounds."

Because no accommodations had been arranged for Miss Nightingale's group of 39 women, they crowded into six small rooms in one of
the hospital's towers. Each room could hold only two with comfort.
Meanwhile the corresponding accommodations in the other tower
were fully occupied by one major. There was no furniture in the dirty
rooms, which were swarming with vermin, and one of them even
contained a long-neglected corpse. The Nightingale nurses wore gray
tweed dresses, gray worsted jackets, plain white caps, short woolen
cloaks, and brown scarves embroidered in red with the words "Scutari
Hospital."

The Barrack Hospital at Scutari was designed to accommodate
1700 patients, but between 3000 and 4000 were tightly packed into it
when Miss Nightingale arrived. There were four miles of beds situated
18 inches apart. The mattresses on the beds, the tiles of the unglazed,
unwashed floor, and even the plaster on the walls were soaked with
liquid excrement. The building was standing in "a sea of sewage."
Lice, maggots, rats, and countless other forms of vermin were crawling
around everywhere. Describing the conditions to Sidney Herbert,
Florence wrote graphically that "the vermin might, if they had but
unity of purpose, carry off the four miles of beds on their backs and
march them into the War Office."

Within 10 days of her arrival, Miss Nightingale had set up a kitchen
for special diets and had rented a house which she converted into a
laundry. After she had hired soldiers' wives to do the washing, clean
linen finally began to appear on the hospital wards. Unable to obtain
any money from the authorities, Miss Nightingale utilized the *Times*
Relief Fund and even her own personal resources to purchase medical
supplies, food, and hospital equipment for virtually an army. Once
satisfied with the improvement in hospital conditions, she initiated
social service work among the soldiers. This program of social welfare,
however, earned her the criticism of the surgeons, who reproached
her for "spoiling the brutes."

In the small room where Florence sat at a plain wooden table
and wrote requests, orders, letters, and reports, there was a narrow
bed, in which she seldom slept. In addition to her heavy administrative
burden, she spent long hours in the wards nursing. Robert Robinson,
a disabled 11-year-old drummer boy from the Sixty-eighth Light
Infantry, served as her personal attendant, delivering messages and

carrying her lamp at night while she went among the crowds of wounded to help during an operation or sit by a dying man.

It was not uncommon for Miss Nightingale to spend eight hours at a time, sometimes on her knees, dressing wounds and comforting the soldiers. At other times she stood for as long as 20 consecutive hours distributing stores, directing her staff, and assisting in operations. On one occasion, when she saw five soldiers laid aside as hopeless cases, she asked permission to care for them. Next morning they were ready to be operated on. "Before she came," one soldier wrote home, "there was cussin' and swearin', but after that it was holy as a church." Another wrote, "What a comfort it was to see her pass even. She would speak to one and nod and smile to as many more, but she could not do it all, you know. We lay there by hundreds, but we could kiss her shadow as it fell, and lay our heads on the pillow again content." "She was all full of life and fun when she talked to us," said another, "especially if a man was a bit downhearted".

Correspondent M.W. Macdonald of the *Times* filed a memorable report on Miss Nightingale's work:

Wherever there is disease in its most dangerous form, and the hand of the despoiler distressingly nigh, there is this incomparable woman (Florence Nightingale) sure to be seen; her benignant presence is an influence for good comfort, even amid the struggles of expiring nature. She is a "ministering angel," without any exaggeration, in these hospitals; and as her slender form glides quietly along each corridor, every poor fellow's face softens with gratitude at the sight of her. When all the medical officers have retired for the night, and silence and darkness have settled down upon those miles of prostrate sick, she may be observed alone, with a little lamp in her hand, making her solitary rounds.

Victorian poet R.N. Cust immortalized Miss Nightingale for the British public in his poem *Scutari Hospital*.

> Moaning in agony,
>   Writhing in pain,
> Fighting the dreadful flight
>   Over again;
> Hearts yearning for home,
>   Yearning in vain,
> Tears over manly cheeks
>   Pouring like rain.
> Thus through the dreary day
>   And dreary night
> Lie England's soldiers
>   After the fight!

Flitting like angels
From bed to bed
Cooling the parched lips
And aching head,
Of the poor mangled limb
Loosening the bands,
Wiping the clammy brows
With tender hands.
Thus through the dreary night
And dreary day
To England's nurses
Hours pass away!

Many a blessing,
Many a prayer,
Burst from rough lips for
Those angels there.
England sends gladly
Her mighty sons,
With implements of war
And battering guns.
And England's daughters
Proudly repair,
In Liberty's battle,
Perils to share!

The difficulties that Miss Nightingale encountered and the prejudices that she had to overcome were enormous. The revolutionary aspect of her work, which did more than just reorganize military hospitals and procure comfort for thousands of wounded soldiers, cannot
be fully measured. As a result of the unprecedented introduction of
women nurses into the British Army, she succeeded in overcoming
age-old prejudices and in elevating the status of all nurses. Probably for
the first time in history, the overwhelming support of public opinion
forced an antagonistic military hierarchy to accept a lady administrator
with extensive authority.

Six months later, in early May, 1855, when conditions at the
Barrack Hospital were reasonably satisfactory, Miss Nightingale jour-
neyed across the Black Sea to the Crimea. Two British hospitals were
located there, both near the seaport of Balaclava. One, the General
Hospital, had been established near the harbor upon the arrival of the
British in September, 1854. The enormous numbers of sick from
cholera, from wounds received at the battles of Balaclava (October 25,

1854) and Inkerman (November 5, 1854), and from the undernourishment and exposure during the winter of 1854-55 had necessitated further accommodations, and a cluster of huts had been erected on the heights near the old Genoese Castle above Balaclava. This complex, which constituted the second hospital, was accordingly called the Castle Hospital.

Accompanying Miss Nightingale to the Crimea was Alexis Soyer, chef at the Reform Club in London, whose task it was to supervise the army's diet. Because he had studied how to cook large quantities of food economically and at the same time serve delicious dishes, he rapidly trained the cooks in the hospital kitchens to prepare excellent meals made strictly with army rations. He invented a special cooking oven, the Soyer boiler, which was used long afterward, and the "Scutari teapot," which could brew tea for half a company of men.

After visiting the front and the hospitals, Florence contracted "Crimean fever" and was taken to the Castle Hospital, where she nearly died. She was evacuated to Scutari, where she narrowly avoided an underhanded effort by Dr. John Hall to ship her directly to England in order to eliminate her "interference" with Medical Staff affairs. Soldiers wept when news of her illness reached them, and all England awaited the outcome in anxious suspense. Within a few weeks she had recovered and resumed her duties at Scutari, but the strain and responsibility of providing nursing care had undermined her health to such an extent that she would never again be able to work with her previous physical vigor.

By the end of the Crimean War, Florence had supervised 125 nurses—a small number by later standards, but large when one considers the oppostion of the Army physicians. When she first arrived at the Barrack Hospital, its mortality rate stood at 60 percent; she left it at a fraction over 1 percent. The general improvement in all British military hospitals is perhaps best indicated by the overall drop in the mortality rate from 42 percent to 2.2 percent. Miss Nightingale's immense courage and indomitable perseverance forced the military authorities to acknowledge that there was a place for women nurses in Army hospitals. In recognition of her services, Queen Victoria presented her with a distinctive brooch bearing the inscription "Blessed are the merciful."

After the Crimean War ended early in 1856, the hospitals were closed one by one, and the nurses returned to England. Miss Nightingale was among the last to leave in July, 1856. Upon her return from the Crimea, she immediately began pursuing the two goals most vital to her:

reform of Army sanitary practices and the establishment of a school for nurses. The latter task was aided by the donation of more than $220,000 by the British public.

When the nurse training school was begun as an experiment at St. Thomas' Hospital in London, the overwhelming majority of London physicians opposed the project. Of the 100 physicians asked, only four favored the school. Most replied that because nurses occupied much the same position as housemaids, they needed little instruction beyond poultice-making, the enforcement of cleanliness, and attention to the patient's personal needs. Miss Nightingale's ill health prevented her from taking charge of the program, but for years she acted as its chief adviser.

In addition to establishing the training school, Miss Nightingale worked to improve the health standards of the British Army. She was determined that the lessons taught by the Crimean War be used to prepare for the future. In order to influence Parliament and the general staff of the British Army, she wrote a study entitled *Notes on Matters Affecting the Health, Efficiency, and Hospital Administration of the British Army* (1858), which was respectfully received by Her Majesty's government. Her *Notes on Hospitals* (1858) was a seminal work, and her *Notes on Nursing* (1859) served for decades as the standard text on nursing. Upon completion of these studies, she undertook the enormous project of investigating sanitary conditions in India.

While the Crimean War caused untold suffering, it also led to one of the greatest humanitarian advances of history: modern military nursing, from which developed professional nursing in general. If it had not been for the horrible conditions in the British hospitals and camps at the beginning of this war, there would have been no nursing reform by Florence Nightingale. Possibly her indomitable spirit would have achieved its goal in some other way, but the frightful things that the "Lady with a Lamp" saw and the heroic things that she did reached the newspapers and gave her the backing of public opinion.

Across the Atlantic, Henry Wadsworth Longfellow paid popular tribute to the "Saint of the Crimea" with his poem *Santa Filomena:*

> *Whene'er a noble deed is wrought,*
> *Whene'er is spoken a noble thought,*
> *Our hearts, in glad surprise,*
> *To higher levels rise.*

The tidal wave of deeper souls
Into our inmost being rolls,
   And lifts us unawares
   Out of all meaner cares.

Honour to those whose words or deeds
Thus help us in our daily needs,
   And by their overflow
   Raise us from what is low!

Thus thought I, as by night I read
Of the great army of the dead,
   The trenches cold and damp,
   The starved and frozen camp—

The wounded from the battle plain,
In dreary hospitals of pain—
   The cheerless corridors,
   The cold and stony floors.

Lo! in that house of misery,
A lady with a lamp I see
   Pass through the glimmering gloom,
   And flit from room to room.

And slow, as in a dream of bliss,
The speechless sufferer turns to kiss
   Her shadow, as it falls
   Upon the darkening walls.

As if a door in heaven should be,
Opened, and then closed suddenly,
   The vision came and went—
   The light shone and was spent.

On England's annals, through the long
Hereafter of her speech and song,
   That light its rays shall cast
   From portals of the past.

A lady with a lamp shall stand
In the great history of the land,
   A noble type of good,
   Heroic womanhood.

Nor even shall be wanting here
The palm, the lily, and the spear,
   The symbols that of yore
   Saint Filomena bore.

Florence Nightingale: Author and Reformer—Rebel?

This popular book (15,000 copies sold in first month after publication), published in 1859, caused a major sensation at the time; many of her personal hygiene suggestions, for example, being considered quite revolutionary by Victorians. Notably, Miss Nightingale did not wish to merely write a manual for nurses. The work was intended for the use of every woman as an "alphabet of household hygiene." In her words, she "meant simply to give hints for thought to women who have personal charge of the health of others." Yet, it is nevertheless an incomparable treatise on nursing praised by contemporaries and moderns alike. In the words of Woodham-Smith, "neither its good sense nor its wit can be dated." Used as a textbook at the pioneering Florence Nightingale School of Nursing, St. Thomas Hospital, it is probably the finest example of her farsightedness on the one hand and her clear association with the age on the other. In this "Conclusion," for example, it can easily be seen why many of its precepts are still valid today: the welfare and the comfort of the patient always coming first, along with the emphasis on plenty of sunlight, proper ventilation and scrupulous cleanliness in the sickroom.

FLORENCE NIGHTINGALE

Notes on Nursing: First Nursing Textbook?

The whole of the preceding remarks apply even more to children and to puerperal woman than to patients in general. They also apply to the nursing of surgical, quite as much as to that of medical cases. Indeed, if it be possible, cases of external injury require such care even more than sick. In surgical wards, one duty of every nurse certainly is *prevention*. Fever, or hospital gangrene, or pyœmia, or purulent discharge of some kind may else supervene. Has she a case of compound fracture, of amputation, or of erysipelas, it may depend very much on how she looks upon the things enumerated in these notes, whether one or other of these hospital diseases attacks her patient or not. If she allows her ward to become filled with the peculiar close fœtid smell, so apt to be produced among surgical cases, especially where there is great suppuration and discharge, she may see a vigorous patient in the prime of life gradually sink and die where, according to all human probability, he ought to have recovered. The surgical nurse must be ever on the watch, ever on her guard, against want of cleanliness, foul air, want of light, and of warmth.

Nevertheless let no one think that because *sanitary* nursing is the subject of these notes, therefore, what may be called the handicraft of nursing is to be undervalued. A patient may be left to bleed to death in a sanitary palace. Another who cannot move himself may die of bed-sores, because the nurse does not know how to change and clean him, while he has every requisite of air, light, and quiet. But nursing, as a handicraft, has not been treated of here for three reasons: 1. That these notes do not pretend to be a manual for nursing, any more than for cooking for the sick; 2. That the writer, who has herself seen more of what may be called surgical nursing, *i.e.* practical manual nursing, than, perhaps any one in Europe, honestly believes that it is impossible to learn it from any book, and that it can only be thorough-ly learnt in the wards of a hospital; and she also honestly believes that the perfection of surgical nursing may be seen practised by the old-fashioned "Sister" of a London hospital, as it can be seen nowhere else in Europe. 3. While thousands die of foul air, &c., who have this surgical nursing to perfection, the converse is comparatively rare.

To revert to children. They are much more susceptible than grown people to all noxious influences. They are affected by the same things, but much more quickly and seriously, viz., by want of fresh air, of proper warmth, want of cleanliness in house, clothes, bedding, or body, by startling noises, improper food, or want of punctuality, by dulness and by want of light, by too much or too little covering in bed, or when up, by want of the spirit of management generally in those in charge of them. One can, therefore, only press the importance, as being yet greater in the case of children, greatest in the case of sick children, of attending to these things.

That which, however, above all, is known to injure children seriously is foul air, and most seriously at night. Keeping the rooms where they sleep tight shut up, is destruction to them. And, if the child's breathing be disordered by disease, a few hours only of such foul air may endanger its life, even where no inconvenience is felt by grown-up persons in the same room.

The following passages, taken out of an excellent "Lecture on Sudden Death in Infancy and Childhood," just published, show the vital importance of careful nursing of children. "In the great majority of instances, when death suddenly befalls the infant or young child it is an *accident*; it is not a necessary result of any disease from which it is suffering."

It may be here added, that it would be very desirable to know how often death is, with adults, "not a necessary, inevitable result of any disease." Omit the word "sudden;" (for *sudden* death is comparatively rare in middle age;) and the sentence is almost equally true for all ages.

The following causes of "accidental" death in sick children are enumerated:—"Sudden noises, which startle—a rapid change of temperature, which chills the surface, though only for a moment—a rude awakening from sleep—or even an over-hasty, or an overfull meal"—"any sudden impression on the nervous system—any hasty alteration of posture—in short, any cause whatever by which the respiratory process may be disturbed."

It may again be added, that, with very weak adult patients, these causes are also (not often "suddenly fatal," it is true, but) very much oftener than is at all generally known, irreparable in their consequences.

Both for children and for adults, both for sick and for well (although more certainly in the case of sick children than in any others), I would here again repeat, the most frequent and most fatal cause of all is sleeping, for even a few hours, much more for weeks and months, in foul air, a condition which, more than any other condition, disturbs the respiratory process, and tends to produce "accidental" death in disease.

I need hardly here repeat the warning against any confusion of ideas between cold and fresh air. You may chill a patient fatally without giving him fresh air at all. And you can quite well, nay, much better, give him fresh air without chilling him. This is the test of a good nurse.

In cases of long recurring faintnesses from disease, for instance, especially disease which affects the organs of breathing, fresh air to the lungs, warmth to the surface, and often (as soon as the patient can swallow) hot drink, these are the right remedies and the only ones. Yet, oftener than not, you see the nurse or mother just reversing this; shutting up every cranny through which fresh air can enter, and leaving the body cold, or perhaps throwing a greater weight of clothes upon it, when already it is generating too little heat.

"Breathing carefully, anxiously, as though respiration were a function which requried all the attention for its performance," is cited as a not unusual state in children, and as one calling for care in all the things enumerated above. That breathing becomes an almost voluntary act, even in grown up patients who are very weak, must often have been remarked.

"Disease having interfered with the perfect accomplishment of the respiratory function, some sudden demand for its complete exercise, issues in the sudden stand-still of the whole machinery," is given as one process:—"life goes out for want of nervous power to keep the vital functions in activity," is given as another, by which "accidental" death is most often brought to pass in infancy.

Also in middle age, both these processes may be seen ending in death, although generally not suddenly. And I have seen, even in middle age, the *"sudden* stand-still" here mentioned, and from the same causes.

To sum up:—the answer to two of the commonest objections urged, one by women themselves, the other by men, against the desirableness of sanitary knowledge, for women, *plus* a caution, comprises the whole argument for the art of nursing.

(1.) It is often said by men, that it is unwise to teach women anything about these laws of health, because they will take to physicking,— that there is a great deal too much of amateur physicking as it is, which is indeed true. One eminent physician told me that he had more calomel given, both at a pinch and for a continuance, by mothers, governesses, and nurses, to children than he had ever heard of a physician prescribing in all his experience. Another says, that women's only idea in medicine is calomel and aperients. This is undeniably too often the case. There is nothing ever seen in any professional practice like the reckless physicking by amateur females.* But this is just what the really experienced and observing nurse does *not* do; she neither physics herself nor others. And to cultivate in things pertaining to health observation and experience in women who are mothers, governesses or nurses, is just the way to do away with amateur physicking, and if the doctors did but know it, to make the nurses obedient to them,—helps to them instead of hindrances. Such education in women would indeed diminish the doctor's work—but

---

*I have known many ladies who, having once obtained a "blue pill" prescription from a physician, gave and took it as a common aperient two or three times a week—with what effect may be supposed. In one case I happened to be the person to inform the physician of it, who substituted from the prescription a comparatively harmless aperient pill. The lady came to me and complained that it "did not suit her half so well."

If women will take or give physic, by far the safest plan is to send for "the doctor" every time—for I have known ladies who both gave and took physic, who would not take the pains to learn the names of the commonest medicines, and confounded, *e.g.*, colocynth with colchicum. This *is* playing with sharp-edged tools "with a vengeance."

There are excellent women who will write to London to their physician that there is much sickness in their neighbourhood in the country, and ask for some prescription from him, which they used to like themselves, and then give it to all their friends and to all their poorer neighbours who will take it. Now, instead of giving medicine, of which you cannot possibly know the exact and proper applications, nor all its consequences, would it not be better if you were to persuade and help your poorer neighbours to remove the dung-hill from before the door, to put in a window which opens, or an Arnott's ventilator, or to cleanse and limewash

no one really believes that doctors wish that there should be more illness, in order to have more work.

(2.) It is often said by women, that they cannot know anything of the laws of health, or what to do to preserve their children's health, because they can know nothing of "Pathology," or cannot "dissect,"—a confusion of ideas which it is hard to attempt to disentangle. Pathology teaches the harm that disease has done. But it teaches nothing more. We know nothing of the principle of health, the positive of which pathology is the negative, except from observation and experience. And nothing but observation and experience will teach us the ways to maintain or to bring back the state of health. It is often thought that medicine is the curative process. It is no such thing; medicine is the surgery of functions, as surgery proper is that of limbs and organs. Neither can do anything but remove obstructions; neither can cure; nature alone cures. Surgery removes the bullet out of the limb, which is an obstruction to cure, but nature heals the wound. So it is with medicine; the function of an organ becomes obstructed; medicine, so far as we know, assists nature to remove the obstruction, but does nothing more. And what nursing has to do in either case, is to put the patient in the best condition for nature to act upon him. Generally, just the contrary is done. You think fresh air, and quiet and cleanliness extravagant, perhaps dangerous, luxuries, which should be given to the patient only when quite convenient, and medicine the *sine qua non*, the panacea. If I have succeeded in any measure in dispelling this illusion, and in showing what true nursing is, and what it is not, my object will have been answered.

---

the cottages? Of these things the benefits are sure. The benefits of the inexperienced administration of medicines are by no means so sure.

Homœopathy has introduced one essential amelioration in the practice of physic by amateur females; for its rules are excellent, its physicking comparatively harmless—the "globule" is the one grain of folly which appears to be necessary to make any good thing acceptable. Let then women, if they will give medicine, give homœopathic medicine. It won't do any harm.

An almost universal error among women is the supposition that everybody *must* have the bowels opened once in every twenty-four hours, or must fly immediately to aperients. The reverse is the conclusion of experience.

This is a doctor's subject, and I will not enter more into it; but will simply repeat, do not go on taking or giving to your children your abominable "courses of aperients," without calling in the doctor.

It is very seldom indeed, that by choosing your diet, you cannot regulate your own bowels; and every woman may watch herself to know what kind of diet will do this; I have known deficiency of meat produce constipation, quite as often as deficiency of vegetables; baker's bread much oftener than either. Home made brown bread will oftener cure it than anything else.

Now for the caution:—

(3.) It seems a commonly received idea among men and even among women themselves that it requires nothing but a disappointment in love, the want of an object, a general disgust, or incapacity for other things, to turn a woman into a good nurse.

This reminds one of the parish where a stupid old man was set to be schoolmaster because he was "past keeping the pigs."

Apply the above receipt for making a good nurse to making a good servant. And the receipt will be found to fail.

Yet popular novelists of recent days have invented ladies disappointed in love or fresh out of the drawing-room turning into the war-hospitals to find their wounded lovers, and when found, forthwith abandoning their sickward for their lover, as might be expected. Yet in the estimation of the authors, these ladies were none the worse for that, but on the contrary were heroines of nursing.

What cruel mistakes are sometimes made by benevolent men and women in matters of business about which they can know nothing and think they know a great deal.

The everyday management of a large ward, let alone of a hospital—the knowing what are the laws of life and death for men, and what the laws of health for wards—(and wards are healthy or unhealthy, mainly according to the knowledge or ignorance of the nurse)—are not these matters of sufficient importance and difficulty to require learning by experience and careful inquiry, just as much as any other art? They do not come by inspiration to the lady disappointed in love, nor to the poor workhouse drudge hard up for a livelihood.

And terrible is the injury which has followed to the sick from such wild notions!

In this respect (and why is it so?), in Roman Catholic countries, both writers and workers are, in theory at least, far before ours. They would never think of such a beginning for a good working Superior or Sister of Charity. And many a Superior has refused to admit a *Postulant* who appeared to have no better "vocation" or reasons for offering herself than these.

It is true *we* make "no vows." But is a "vow" necessary to convince us that the true spirit for learning any art, most especially an art of charity, aright, is not a disgust to everything or something else? Do we really place the love of our kind (and of nursing, as one branch of it) so low as this? What would the Mère Angélique of Port Royal, what would our own Mrs. Fry have said to this?

NOTE.—I would earnestly ask my sisters to keep clear of both the jargons now current everywhere (for they *are* equally jargous); of the jargon, namely, about the "rights" of women, which urges women to do all that men do, including the medical and other professions, merely because men do it, and without regard to whether this *is* the best that women can do; and of the jargon which urges women to do nothing that men do, merely because they are women, and should be "recalled to a sense of their duty as women," and because "this is women's work," and "that is men's," and "these are things which women should not do," which is all assertion, and nothing more. Surely woman should bring the best she has, *whatever* that is, to the work of God's world, without attending to either of these cries. For what are they, both of them, the one *just* as much as the other, but listening to the "what people will say," to opinion, to the "voices from without?" And as a wise man has said, no one has ever done anything great or useful by listening to the voices from without.

You do not want the effect of your good things to be, "How wonderful for a *woman!*" nor would you be deterred from good things by hearing it said, "Yes, but she ought not to have done this, because it is not suitable for a woman." But you want to do the thing that is good, whether it is "suitable for a woman" or not.

It does not make a thing good, that it is remarkable that a woman should have been able to do it. Neither does it make a thing bad, which would have been good had a man done it, that it has been done by a woman.

Oh, leave these jargons, and go your way straight to God's work, in simplicity and singleness of heart.

Lytton Strachey, well-known critic and literary figure in the early twentieth century (leader of the celebrated "Bloomsbury" circle), was often praised for his gift of vivid historical biography. His stated purpose was to "lay bare the facts of some cases . . . dispassionately, impartially and without ulterior intentions." It must not be forgotten, however, that, in the process, he was rebelling against the beliefs and habits of orthodox middle-class Victorianism. Filled with acid irony, biting satire and savage wit, his *Eminent Victorians* makes four of the age's heroes (Cardinal Henry Manning, Dr. Thomas Arnold, General Charles Gordon and Florence Nightingale) seem almost too human. In the words of Joseph Wood Krutch, "with every word a reputation dies under the quiet deadliness of his rapier." In this excerpt, for example, Strachey rejects the popular conception of the "saintly, self-sacrificing woman, the delicate maiden of a high degree"; describing her instead as a woman moving under a different stress and impetus, driven by the "demon who possessed her." Her many supporters dismissed him as an "iconoclast" and yet, while certainly harsh, the portrait has nonetheless shaped all later understanding of her personality.

G. LYTTON STRACHEY (1880-1932)

Florence Nightingale: A Woman Possessed?

I

Every one knows the popular conception of Florence Nightingale. The saintly, self-sacrificing woman, the delicate maiden of high degree who threw aside the pleasures of a life of ease to succour the afflicted, the Lady with the Lamp, gliding through the horrors of the hospital at Scutari, and consecrating with the radiance of her goodness the dying soldier's couch—the vision is familiar to all. But the truth was different. The Miss Nightingale of fact was not as facile fancy painted her. She worked in another fashion, and towards another end; she moved under the stress of an impetus which finds no place in the popular imagination. A Demon possessed her. Now demons, whatever else they may be, are full of interest. And so it happens that in the real Miss Nightingale there was more that was interesting than in the legendary one; there was also less that was agreeable. . . .

III

The name of Florence Nightingale lives in the memory of the world by virtue of the lurid and heroic adventure of the Crimea. Had she died—as she nearly did—upon her return to England, her reputation would hardly have been different; her legend would have come down to us almost as we know it to-day—that gentle vision of female virtue which first took shape before the adoring eyes of the sick soldiers at Scutari. Yet, as a matter of fact, she lived for more than half a century after the Crimean War; and during the greater part of that long period all the energy and all the devotion of her extraordinary nature were working at their highest pitch. What she accomplished in those years of unknown labour could, indeed, hardly have been more glorious than her Crimean triumphs; but it was certainly more important. The true history was far stranger even than the myth. In Miss Nightingale's own eyes the adventure of the Crimea was a mere incident—scarcely more than a useful stepping-stone in her career. It was the fulcrum with which she hoped to move the world; but it was only the fulcrum. For more than a generation she was to sit in secret, working her lever: and her real life began at the very moment when, in the popular imagination, it had ended.

She arrived in England in a shattered state of health. The hardships and the ceaseless effort of the last two years had undermined her nervous system; her heart was pronounced to be affected; she suffered constantly from fainting-fits and terrible attacks of utter physical prostration. The doctors declared that one thing alone would save her—a complete and prolonged rest. But that was also the one thing with which she would have nothing to do. She had never been in the habit of resting; why should she begin now? Now, when her opportunity had come at last; now, when the iron was hot, and it was time to strike? No; she had work to do; and, come what might, she would do it. The doctors protested in vain; in vain her family lamented and entreated, in vain her friends pointed out to her the madness of such a course. Madness? Mad-possessed—perhaps she was. A demoniac frenzy had seized upon her. As she lay upon her sofa, gasping, she devoured blue-books, dictated letters, and, in the intervals of her palpitations, cracked her febrile jokes. For months at a stretch she never left her bed. For years she was in daily expectation of death. But she would not rest. At this rate, the doctors assured her, even if she did not die, she would become an invalid for life. She could not help that; there was the work to be done; and, as for rest, very likely she might rest . . . when she had done it.

Wherever she went, in London or in the country, in the hills of Derbyshire, or among the rhododendrons at Embley, she was haunted by a ghost. It was the spectre of Scutari—the hideous vision of the organisation of a military hospital. She would lay that phantom, or she would perish. The whole system of the Army Medical Department, the education of the Medical Officer, the regulations of hospital procedure . . . *rest*? How could she rest while these things were as they were, while, if the like necessity were to arise again, the like results would follow? And, even in peace and at home, what was the sanitary condition of the Army? The mortality in the barracks was, she found, nearly double the mortality in civil life. 'You might as well take 1,100 men every year out upon Salisbury Plain and shoot them,' she said. After inspecting the hospitals at Chatham, she smiled grimly. 'Yes, this is one more symptom of the system which, in the Crimea, put to death 16,000 men.' Scutari had given her knowledge; and it had given her power too: her enormous reputation was at her back—an incalculable force. Other work, other duties, might lie before her; but the most urgent, the most obvious, of all was to look to the health of the Army.

One of her very first steps was to take advantage of the invitation which Queen Victoria had sent her to the Crimea, together with the commemorative brooch. Within a few weeks of her return she visited Balmoral, and had several interviews with both the Queen and the Prince Consort. 'She put before us,' wrote the Prince in his diary, 'all the defects of our present military hospital system, and the reforms that are needed.' She related 'the whole story' of her experiences in the East; and, in addition, she managed to have some long and confidential talks with His Royal Highness on metaphysics and religion. The impression which she created was excellent. 'Sie gefällt uns sehr,' noted the Prince, 'ist sehr bescheiden.' Her Majesty's comment was different—'Such a *head*! I wish we had her at the War Office.'

But Miss Nightingale was not at the War Office, and for a very simple reason: she was a woman. Lord Panmure, however, *was* (though indeed the reason for that was not quite so simple); and it was upon Lord Panmure that the issue of Miss Nightingale's efforts for reform must primarily depend. That burly Scottish nobleman had not, in spite of his most earnest endeavours, had a very easy time of it as Secretary of State for War. He had come into office in the middle of the Sebastopol Campaign, and had felt himself very well fitted for the position, since he had acquired in former days an inside knowledge of the Army—as a

Captain of Hussars. It was this inside knowledge which had enabled him to inform Miss Nightingale with such authority that 'the British soldier is not a remitting animal.' And perhaps it was this same consciousness of a command of his subject which had impelled him to write a dispatch to Lord Raglan, blandly informing the Commander-in-Chief in the Field just how he was neglecting his duties, and pointing out to him that if he would only try he really might do a little better next time. Lord Raglan's reply, calculated as it was to make its recipient sink into the earth, did not quite have that effect upon Lord Panmure, who, whatever might have been his faults, had never been accused of being supersensitive. However, he allowed the matter to drop; and a little later Lord Raglan died—worn out, some people said, by work and anxiety. He was succeeded by an excellent red-nosed old gentleman, General Simpson, whom nobody has ever heard of, and who took Sebastopol. But Lord Panmure's relations with him were hardly more satisfactory than his relations with Lord Raglan; for, while Lord Raglan had been too independent, poor General Simpson erred in the opposite direction, perpetually asked advice, suffered from lumbago, doubted, his nose growing daily redder and redder, whether he was fit for his post, and, by alternate mails, sent in and withdrew his resignation. Then, too, both the General and the Minister suffered acutely from that distressingly useful new invention, the electric telegraph. On one occasion General Simpson felt obliged actually to expostulate. 'I think, my Lord,' he wrote, 'that some telegraphic messages reach us that cannot be sent under due authority, and are perhaps unknown to you, although under the protection of your Lordship's name. For instance, I was called up last night, a dragoon having come express with a telegraphic message in these words, "Lord Panmure to General Simpson—Captain Jarvis has been bitten by a centipede. How is he now?"' General Simpson might have put up with this, though to be sure it did seem 'rather too trifling an affair to call for a dragoon to ride a couple of miles in the dark that he may knock up the Commander of the Army out of the very small allowance of sleep permitted him'; but what was really more than he could bear was to find 'upon sending in the morning another mounted dragoon to inquire after Captain Jarvis, four miles off, that he never has been bitten at all, but has had a boil, from which he is fast recovering'. But Lord Panmure had troubles of his own. His favourite nephew, Captain Dowbiggin, was at the front, and to one of his telegrams to the Commander-in-Chief the Minister had taken occasion to append the following carefully qualified sentence—'I recommend Dowbiggin to your notice, should you have a vacancy, and

if he is fit.' Unfortunately, in those early days, it was left to the discretion of the telegraphist to compress the messages which passed
through his hands; so that the result was that Lord Panmure's delicate
appeal reached its destination in the laconic form of 'Look after Dowb'.
The Headquarters Staff were at first extremely puzzled; they were at
last extremely amused. The story spread; and 'Look after Dowb'
remained for many years the familiar formula for describing official
hints in favour of deserving nephews.

And now that all this was over, now that Sebastopol had been,
somehow or another, taken, now that peace was, somehow or another,
made, now that the troubles of office might surely be expected to be at
an end at last—here was Miss Nightingale breaking in upon the scene,
with her talk about the state of the hospitals and the necessity for
sanitary reform. It was most irksome; and Lord Panmure almost began
to wish that he was engaged upon some more congenial occupation—
discussing, perhaps, the constitution of the Free Church of Scotland—
a question in which he was profoundly interested. But no; duty was
paramount; and he set himself, with a sigh of resignation, to the task
of doing as little of it as he possibly could.

'The Bison' his friends called him; and the name fitted both his
physical demeanour and his habit of mind. That large low head seemed
to have been created for butting rather than for anything else. There he
stood, four-square and menacing, in the doorway of reform; and it
remained to be seen whether the bulky mass, upon whose solid hide
even the barbed arrows of Lord Raglan's scorn had made no mark,
would prove amenable to the pressure of Miss Nightingale. Nor was
he alone in the doorway. There loomed behind him the whole phalanx
of professional conservatism, the stubborn supporters of the out-of-date,
the worshippers and the victims of War Office routine. Among these it
was only natural that Dr. Andrew Smith, the head of the Army Medical
Department, should have been pre-eminent—Dr. Andrew Smith, who
had assured Miss Nightingale before she left England that 'nothing was
wanted at Scutari'. Such were her opponents; but she too was not without allies. She had gained the ear of Royalty—which was something;
at any moment that she pleased she could gain the ear of the public—
which was a great deal. She had a host of admirers and friends; and—
to say nothing of her personal qualities—her knowledge, her tenacity,
her tact—she possessed, too, one advantage which then, far more even
than now, carried an immense weight—she belonged to the highest
circle of society. She moved naturally among Peers and Cabinet Members—she was one of their own set; and in those days their set was a

very narrow one. What kind of attention would such persons have paid to some middle-class woman with whom they were not acquainted, who possessed great experience of Army nursing and had decided views upon hospital reform? They would have politely ignored her; but it was impossible to ignore Florence Nightingale. When she spoke, they were obliged to listen; and, when they had once begun to do that—what might not follow? She knew her power, and she used it. She supported her weightiest minutes with familiar witty little ones. The Bison began to look grave. It might be difficult—it might be damned difficult—to put down one's head against the white hand of a lady.

Of Miss Nightingale's friends, the most important was Sidney Herbert. He was a man upon whom the good fairies seemed to have showered, as he lay in his cradle, all their most enviable goods. Well born, handsome, rich, the master of Wilton—one of those great country-houses, clothed with the glamour of a historic past, which are the peculiar glory of England—he possessed, besides all these advantages, so charming, so lively, so gentle a disposition that no one who had once come near him could ever be his enemy. He was, in fact, a man of whom it was difficult not to say that he was a perfect English gentleman. For his virtues were equal even to his good fortune. He was reigious—deeply religious: 'I am more and more convinced every day,' he wrote, when he had been for some years a Cabinet Minister, 'that in politics, as in everything else, nothing can be right which is not in accordance with the spirit of the Gospel.' No one was more unselfish; he was charitable and benevolent to a remarkable degree; and he devoted the whole of his life with an unwavering conscientiousness to the public service. With such a character, with such opportunities, what high hopes must have danced before him, what radiant visions of accomplished duties, of ever-increasing usefulness, of beneficent power, of the consciousness of disinterested success! Some of those hopes and visions were, indeed, realised; but, in the end, the career of Sidney Herbert seemed to show that, with all their generosity, there was some gift or other—what was it?—some essential gift—which the good fairies had withheld, and that even the qualities of a perfect English gentleman may be no safeguard against anguish, humiliation, and defeat.

That career would certainly have been very different if he had never known Miss Nightingale. The alliance between them which had begun with her appointment to Scutari, which had grown closer and closer while the war lasted, developed, after her return, into one of the most extraordinary of friendships. It was the friendship of a man and a woman intimately bound together by their devotion to a public cause; mutual affection, of course, played a part it it, but it was an incidental part; the whole soul of the relationship was a community of work. Perhaps out of England such an intimacy could hardly have existed—an intimacy so utterly untinctured not only by passion itself but by the suspicion of it. For years Sidney Herbert saw Miss Nightingale almost daily, for long hours together, corresponding with her incessantly when they were apart; and the tongue of scandal was silent; and one of the most devoted of her admirers was his wife. But what made the connection still more remarkable was the way in which the parts that were played in it were divided between the two. The man who acts, decides, and achieves; the woman who encourages, applauds, and—from a distance—inspires: the combination is common enough; but Miss Nightingale was neither an Aspasia nor an Egeria. In her case it is almost true to say that the roles were reversed; the qualities of pliancy and sympathy fell to the man, those of command and initiative to the woman. There was one thing only which Miss Nightingale lacked in her equipment for public life; she had not—she never could have—the public power and authority which belong to the successful politician. That power and authority Sidney Herbert possessed; that fact was obvious, and the conclusions no less so: it was through the man that the woman must work her will. She took hold of him, taught him, shaped him, absorbed him, dominated him through and through. He did not resist—he did not wish to resist; his natural inclination lay along the same path as hers; only that terrific personality swept him forward at her own fierce pace and with her own relentless stride. Swept him—where to? Ah! Why had he ever known Miss Nightingale? If Lord Panmure was a bison, Sidney Herbert, no doubt, was a stag—a comely, gallant creature springing through the forest; but the forest is a dangerous place. One has the image of those wide eyes fascinated suddenly by something feline, something strong; there is a pause; and then the tigress has her claws in the quivering haunches; and then——!

Besides Sidney Herbert, she had other friends who, in a more restricted sphere, were hardly less essential to her. If, in her condition of bodily collapse, she were to accomplish what she was determined that she should accomplish, the attentions and the services of others would be absolutely indispensable. Helpers and servers she must have; and accordingly there was soon formed about her a little group of devoted disciples upon whose affections and energies she could implicitly rely. Devoted, indeed, these disciples were, in no ordinary sense of the term; for certainly she was no light task-mistress, and he who set out to be of use to Miss Nightingale was apt to find, before he had gone very far, that he was in truth being made use of in good earnest—to the very limit of his endurance and his capacity. Perhaps, even beyond those limits; why not? Was she asking of others more than she was giving herself? Let them look at her lying there pale and breathless on the couch; could it be said that she spared herself? Why, then, should she spare others? And it was not for her own sake that she made these claims. For her own sake, indeed! No! They all knew it! it was for the sake of the work. And so the little band, bound body and soul in that strange servitude, laboured on ungrudgingly. Among the most faithful was her 'Aunt Mai', her father's sister, who from the earliest days had stood beside her, who had helped her to escape from the thraldom of family life, who had been with her at Scutari, and who now acted almost the part of a mother to her, watching over her with infinite care in all the movements and uncertainties which her state of health involved. Another constant attendant was her brother-in-law, Sir Harry Verney, whom she found particularly valuable in parliamentary affairs. Arthur Clough, the poet, also a connection by marriage, she used in other ways. Ever since he had lost his faith at the time of the Oxford Movement, Clough had passed his life in a condition of considerable uneasiness, which was increased rather than diminished by the practice of poetry. Unable to decide upon the purpose of an existence whose savour had fled together with his belief in the Resurrection, his spirits lowered still further by ill-health, and his income not all that it should be, he had determined to seek the solution of his difficulties in the United States of America. But, even there, the solution was not forthcoming; and when, a little later, he was offered a post in a government department at home, he accepted it, came to live in London, and immediately fell under the influence of Miss Nightingale. Though the purpose of existence might be still uncertain and its nature still unsavoury, here, at any rate, under the eye of this inspired woman, was something real, something earnest: his only doubt was—could he be of any use? Certainly he could. There were a great number of miscellaneous little jobs which there was nobody handy to do. For instance, when Miss Nightingale was travelling, there were the railway-tickets to be taken; and there were proof-sheets to be corrected; and then there were parcels to be done up in brown paper. and carried to the post. Certainly he could be useful. And so, upon such occupations as these, Arthur Clough was set to work. 'This that I see, is not all,' he comforted himself by reflecting, 'and this that I do is but little; nevertheless it is good, though there is better than it.'

As time went on, her 'Cabinet', as she called it, grew larger. Officials with whom her work brought her into touch and who sympathised with her objects, were pressed into her service; and old friends of the Crimean days gathered round her when they returned to England. Among these the most indefatigable was Dr. Sutherland, a sanitary expert, who for more than thirty years acted as her confidential private secretary, and surrendered to her purposes literally the whole of his life. Thus sustained and assisted, thus slaved for and adored, she prepared to beard the Bison.

Two facts soon emerged, and all that followed turned upon them. It became clear, in the first place, that that imposing mass was not immovable, and, in the second, that its movement, when it did move, would be exceeding slow. The Bison was no match for the Lady. It was in vain that he put down his head and planted his feet in the earth; he could not withstand her; the white hand forced him back. But the process was an extraordinarily gradual one. Dr. Andrew Smith and all his War Office phalanx stood behind, blocking the way; the poor Bison groaned inwardly, and cast a wistful eye towards the happy pastures of the Free Church of Scotland; then slowly, with infinite reluctance, step by step, he retreated, disputing every inch of the ground.

The first great measure, which, supported as it was by the Queen, the Cabinet, and the united opinion of the country, it was impossible to resist, was the appointment of a Royal Commission to report upon the health of the Army. The question of the composition of the Commission then immediately arose; and it was over this matter that the first hand-to-hand encounter between Lord Panmure and Miss Nightingale took place. They met, and Miss Nightingale was victorious; Sidney Herbert was appointed Chairman; and, in the end, the only member of the Commission opposed to her views was Dr. Andrew Smith. During the interview, Miss Nightingale made an important discovery: she found that 'the Bison was bullyable'—the hide was the hide of a Mexican buffalo, but the spirit was the spirit of an Alderney calf. And there was one thing above all others which the huge creature dreaded—an appeal to public opinion. The faintest hint of such a terrible eventuality made his heart dissolve within him; he would agree to anything—he would cut short his grouse-shooting—he would make a speech in the House of Lords—he would even overrule Dr. Andrew Smith—rather than that. Miss Nightingale held the fearful threat in reserve—she would speak out what she knew; she would publish the truth to the whole world, and let the whole world judge between them. With supreme skill, she kept this sword of Damocles poised above the Bison's head, and more than once she was actually on the point of really dropping it. For his recalcitrancy grew and grew. The personnel of the Commission once determined upon, there was a struggle, which lasted for six months, over the nature of its powers. Was it to be an efficient body, armed with the right of full inquiry and wide examination, or was it to be a polite official contrivance for exonerating Dr. Andrew Smith? The War Office phalanx closed its ranks, and fought tooth and nail; but it was defeated: the Bison was bullyable. 'Three months from this day,' Miss Nightingale had written at last, 'I publish my experience of the Crimean Campaign, and my suggestions for improvement, unless there has been a fair and tangible pledge by that time for reform.' Who could face that?

And, if the need came, she meant to be as good as her word. For she had now determined, whatever might be the fate of the Commission, to draw up her own report upon the questions at issue. The labour involved was enormous; her health was almost desperate; but she did not flinch, and after six months of incredible industry she had put together and written with her own hand her *Notes affecting the Health, Efficiency, and Hospital Administration of the British Army.* This extraordinary composition, filling more than 800 closely printed pages, laying down vast principles of far-reaching reform, discussing the minutest details of a multitude of controversial subjects, containing an enormous mass of information of the most varied kinds—military, statistical, sanitary, architectural—was never given to the public, for the need never came; but it formed the basis of the Report of the Royal Commission; and it remains to this day the leading authority on the medical administration of armies.

Before it had been completed the struggle over the powers of the Commission had been brought to a victorious close. Lord Panmure had given way once more; he had immediately hurried to the Queen to obtain her consent; and only then, when Her Majesty's initials had been irrevocably affixed to the fatal document, did he dare tell Dr. Andrew Smith what he had done. The Commission met, and another immense load fell upon Miss Nightingale's shoulders. To-day she would, of course, have been one of the Commission herself; but at that time the idea of a woman appearing in such a capacity was unheard of; and no one even suggested the possibility of Miss Nightingale's doing so. The result was that she was obliged to remain behind the scenes throughout, to coach Sidney Herbert in private at every important juncture,

and to convey to him and to her other friends upon the Commission
the vast funds of her expert knowledge—so essential in the examination
of witnesses—by means of innumerable consultations, letters, and memoranda. It was even doubtful whether the proprieties would admit of
her giving evidence; and at last, as a compromise, her modesty only
allowed her to do so in the form of written answers to written questions. At length the grand affair was finished. The Commission's Report,
embodying almost word for word the suggestions of Miss Nightingale,
was drawn up by Sidney Herbert. Only one question remained to be
answered—would anything, after all be done? Or would the Royal Commission, like so many other Royal Commissions before and since, turn
out to have achieved nothing but the concoction of a very fat blue-
book on a very high shelf?

And so the last and the deadliest struggle with the Bison began.
Six months had been spent in coercing him into granting the Commission effective powers; six more months were occupied by the
work of the Commission; and now yet another six were to pass in
extorting from him the means whereby the recommendations of the
Commission might be actually carried out. But, in the end, the thing
was done. Miss Nightingale seemed, indeed, during these months, to
be upon the very brink of death. Accompanied by the faithful Aunt
Mai, she moved from place to place—to Hampstead, to Highgate, to
Derbyshire, to Malvern—in what appeared to be a last desperate effort
to find health somewhere; but she carried that with her which made
health impossible. Her desire for work could now scarcely be distinguished from mania. At one moment she was writing a 'last letter' to
Sidney Herbert; at the next she was offering to go out to India to nurse
the sufferers in the Mutiny. When Dr Sutherland wrote, imploring her
to take a holiday, she raved. Rest!—'I am lying without my head, without my claws, and you all peck at me. It is *de rigueur, d'obligation*, like
the saying something to one's hat, when one goes into church, to say to
me all that has been said to me 110 times a day during the last three
months. It is the *obbligato* on the violin, and the twelve violins all
practise it together, like the clocks striking twelve o'clock at night all
over London, till I say like Xavier de Maistre, *Assez, je le sais, je ne le
sais que trop*. I am not a penitent; but you are like the R.C. confessor,
who says what is *de rigueur....*' Her wits began to turn, and there was
no holding her. She worked like a slave in a mine. She began to believe,
as she had begun to believe at Scutari, that none of her fellow-workers
had their hearts in the business; if they had, why did they not work as
she did? She could only see slackness and stupidity around her. Dr
Sutherland, of course, was grotesquely muddle-headed; and Arthur

Clough incurably lazy. Even Sidney Herbert . . . oh yes, he had simplicity and candour and quickness of perception, no doubt; but he was
an eclectic; and what could one hope for from a man who went away
to fish in Ireland just when the Bison most needed bullying? As for the
Bison himself he had fled to Scotland, where he remained buried for
many months. The fate of the vital recommendation in the Commission's Report—the appointment of four Sub-Commissions charged with
the duty of determining upon the details of the proposed reforms and
of putting them into execution—still hung in the balance. The Bison
consented to everything; and then, on a flying visit to London, withdrew his consent and hastily returned to Scotland. Then for many
weeks all business was suspended; he had gout—gout in the hands, so
that he could not write. 'His gout was always handy,' remarked Miss
Nightingale. But eventually it was clear even to the Bison that the
game was up, and the inevitable surrender came.

There was, however, one point in which he triumphed over Miss
Nightingale. The building of Netley Hospital had been begun, under his
orders, before her return to England. Soon after her arrival she examined
the plans, and found that they reproduced all the worst faults of an
out-of-date and mischievous system of hospital construction. She therefore urged that the matter should be reconsidered, and in the meantime the building stopped. But the Bison was obdurate; it would be very
expensive, and in any case it was too late. Unable to make any impression on him, and convinced of the extreme importance of the question,
she determined to appeal to a higher authority. Lord Palmerston was
Prime Minister; she had known him from her childhood; he was a near
neighbour of her father's in the New Forest. She went down to the New
Forest, armed with the plans of the proposed hospital and all the rele-
vant information, stayed the night at Lord Palmerston's house, and
convinced him of the necessity of rebuilding Netley. 'It seems to me,'
Lord Palmerston wrote to Lord Panmure, 'that at Netley all consideration of what would best tend to the comfort and recovery of the patients
has been sacrificed to the vanity of the architect, whose sole object has
been to make a building which should cut a dash when looked at from
the Southampton river. . . . Pray, therefore, stop all further progress in
the work until the matter can be duly considered.' But the Bison was
not to be moved by one peremptory letter, even if it was from the
Prime Minister. He put forth all his powers of procrastination, Lord
Palmerston lost interest in the subject, and so the chief military hospital
in England was triumphantly completed on insanitary principles, with
unventilated rooms, and with all the patients' windows facing north-east.

But now the time had come when the Bison was to trouble and to be troubled no more. A vote in the House of Commons brought about the fall of Lord Palmerston's Government, and Lord Panmure found himself at liberty to devote the rest of his life to the Free Church of Scotland. After a brief interval, Sidney Herbert became Secretary of State for War. Great was the jubilation in the Nightingale Cabinet: the day of achievement had dawned at last. The next two and a half years (1859-61) saw the introduction of the whole system of reforms for which Miss Nightingale had been struggling so fiercely—reforms which make Sidney Herbert's tenure of power at the War Office an important epoch in the history of the British Army. The four Sub-Commissions, firmly established under the immediate control of the Minister, and urged forward by the relentless perseverance of Miss Nightingale, set to work with a will. The barracks and the hospitals were remodelled; they were properly ventilated and warmed and lighted for the first time; they were given a water supply which actually supplied water, and kitchens where, strange to say, it was possible to cook. Then the great question of the Purveyor—the portentous functionary whose powers and whose lack of powers had weighed like a nightmare upon Scutari—was taken in hand, and new regulations were laid down, accurately defining his responsibilities and his duties. One Sub-Commission reorganised the medical statistics of the Army. Another established—in spite of the last convulsive efforts of the Department—an Army Medical School. Finally the Army Medical Department itself was completely reorganised; an administrative code was drawn up; and the great and novel principle was established that it was as much a part of the duty of the authorities to look after the soldier's health as to look after his sickness. Besides this, it was at last officially admitted that he had a moral and intellectual side. Coffee-rooms and reading-rooms, gymnasiums and workshops were instituted. A new era did in truth appear to have begun. Already by 1861 the mortality in the Army had decreased by one-half since the days of the Crimea. It was no wonder that even vaster possibilities began now to open out before Miss Nightingale. One thing was still needed to complete and to assure her triumphs. The Army Medical Department was indeed reorganised; but the great central machine was still untouched. The War Office itself—!—If she could remould *that* nearer to her heart's desire—there indeed would be a victory! And until that final act was accomplished, how could she be certain that all the rest of her achievements might not, by some capricious turn of Fortune's wheel—a change of Ministry, perhaps, replacing Sidney Herbert by some puppet of the permanent official gang—be swept to limbo in a moment?

Meanwhile, still ravenous for more and yet more work, her activities had branched out into new directions. The Army in India claimed her attention. A Sanitary Commission, appointed at her suggestion, and working under her auspices, did for our troops there what the four Sub-Commissions were doing for those at home. At the same time, these very years which saw her laying the foundations of the whole modern system of medical work in the Army, saw her also beginning to bring her knowledge, her influence, and her activity into the service of the country at large. Her *Notes on Hospitals* (1859) revolutionised the theory of hospital construction and hospital management. She was immediately recognised as the leading expert upon all the questions involved; her advice flowed unceasingly and in all directions, so that there is no great hospital to-day which does not bear upon it the impress of her mind. Nor was this all. With the opening of the Nightingale Training School for Nurses at St Thomas's Hospital (1860), she became the founder of modern nursing.

But a terrible crisis was now fast approaching. Sidney Herbert had consented to undertake the root and branch reform of the War Office. He had sallied forth into that tropical jungle of festooned obstructiveness, of intertwisted irresponsibilities, of crouching prejudices, of abuses grown stiff and rigid with antiquity, which for so many years to come was destined to lure reforming Ministers to their doom. 'The War Office,' said Miss Nightingale, 'is a very slow office, an enormously expensive office, and one in which the Minister's intentions can be entirely negatived by all his sub-departments, and those of each of the sub-departments by every other.' It was true; and, of course, at the first rumour of a change, the old phalanx of reaction was bristling with its accustomed spears. At its head stood no longer Dr Andrew Smith, who, some time since, had followed the Bison into outer darkness, but a yet more formidable figure, the Permanent Under-Secretary himself, Sir Benjamin Hawes—Ben Hawes the Nightingale Cabinet irreverently dubbed him—a man remarkable even among civil servants for adroitness in baffling inconvenient inquiries, resource in raising false issues, and, in short, a consummate command of all the arts of officially sticking in the mud. 'Our scheme will probably result in Ben Hawes's resignation,' Miss Nightingale said; 'and that is another of its advantages.' Ben Hawes himself, however, did not quite see it in that light. He set himself to resist the wishes of the Minister by every means in his power. The struggle was long and desperate; and, as it proceeded, it gradually became evident to Miss Nightingale that something was the matter with Sidney Herbert. What was it? His health, never very strong, was, he said, in danger of collapsing under the strain of his work. But, after all, what is illness, when there is a War Office to be reorganised? Then he began to talk of retiring altogether from public life. The doctors were consulted, and declared that, above all things, what was necessary was rest. Rest! She grew seriously alarmed. Was it possible that, at the last moment, the crowning wreath of victory was to be snatched from her grasp? She was not to be put aside by doctors; they were talking nonsense; the necessary thing was not rest but the reform of the War Office; and, besides, she knew very well from her own case what one could do even when one was on the point of death. She expostulated vehemently, passionately; the goal was so near, so very near; he could not turn back now! At any rate, he could not resist Miss Nightingale. A compromise was arranged. Very reluctantly, he exchanged the turmoil of the House of Commons for the dignity of the House of Lords, and he remained at the War Office. She was delighted. 'One fight more, the best and the last,' she said.

For several more months the fight did indeed go on. But the strain upon him was greater even than she perhaps could realise. Besides the intestine war in his office, he had to face a constant battle in the Cabinet with Mr Gladstone—a more redoubtable antagonist even than Ben Hawes—over the estimates. His health grew worse and worse. He was attacked by fainting-fits; and there were some days when he could only just keep himself going by gulps of brandy. Miss Nightingale spurred him forward with her encouragements and her admonitions, her zeal and her example. But at last his spirit began to sink as well as his body. He could no longer hope; he could no longer desire; it was useless, all useless; it was utterly impossible. He had failed. The dreadful moment came when the truth was forced upon him: he would never be able to reform the War Office. But a yet more dreadful moment lay behind; he must go to Miss Nightingale and tell her that he was a failure, a beaten man.

'Blessed are the merciful!' What strange ironic prescience had led Prince Albert, in the simplicity of his heart, to choose that motto for the Crimean brooch? The words hold a double lesson; and, alas! when she brought herself to realise at length what was indeed the fact and what there was no helping, it was not in mercy that she turned upon her old friend. 'Beaten!' she exclaimed. 'Can't you see that you've simply thrown away the game? And with all the winning cards in your hands! And so noble a game! Sidney Herbert beaten! And beaten by Ben Hawes! It is a worse disgrace . . .' her full rage burst out at last, ' . . . a worse disgrace than the hospitals at Scutari.'

He dragged himself away from her, dragged himself to Spa, hoping vainly for a return to health, and then, despairing, back again to England, to Wilton, to the majestic house standing there resplendent in the summer sunshine, among the great cedars which had lent their shade to Sir Philip Sidney, and all those familiar, darling haunts of beauty which he loved, each one of them, 'as if they were persons'; and at Wilton he died. After having received the Eucharist, he had become perfectly calm; then, almost unconscious, his lips were seen to be moving. Those about him bent down. 'Poor Florence! Poor Florence!' they just caught. ' . . . Our joint work . . . unfinished . . . tried to do . . .' and they could hear no more.

When the onward rush of a powerful spirit sweeps a weaker one to its destruction, the commonplaces of the moral judgement are better left unmade. If Miss Nightingale had been less ruthless, Sidney Herbert would not have perished; but then, she would not have been Miss Nightingale. The force that created was the force that destroyed. It was her Demon that was responsible. When the fatal news reached her, she was overcome by agony. In the revulsion of her feelings, she made a worship of the dead man's memory; and the facile instrument which had broken in her hand she spoke of for ever after as her 'Master'. Then, almost at the same moment, another blow fell on her. Arthur Clough, worn out by labours very different from those of Sidney Herbert, died too: never more would he tie up her parcels. And yet a third disaster followed. The faithful Aunt Mai did not; to be sure, die; no, she did something almost worse: she left Miss Nightingale. She was growing old, and she felt that she had closer and more imperative duties with her own family. Her niece could hardly forgive her. She poured out, in one of her enormous letters, a passionate diatribe upon the faithlessness, the lack of sympathy, the stupidity, the ineptitude of women. Her doctrines had taken no hold among them; she had never known one who had *appris à apprendre*; she could not even get a woman secretary; 'they don't know the names of the Cabinet Ministers—they don't know which of the Churches has Bishops and which not'. As for the spirit of self-sacrifice, well—Sidney Herbert and Arthur Clough were men, and they indeed had shown their devotion; but women——! She would mount three widow's caps 'for a sign'. The first two would be for Clough and for her Master; but the third—'the biggest widow's cap of all'—would be for Aunt Mai. She did well to be angry; she was deserted in her hour of need; and, after all, could she be sure that even the male sex was so impeccable? There was Dr Sutherland, bungling as usual. Perhaps even he intended to go off, one of these

days, too? She gave him a look, and he shivered in his shoes. No!—
she grinned sardonically; she would always have Dr Sutherland. And
then she reflected that there was one thing more that she would always have—her work.

In honor of the centenary of Florence Nightingale's work in the Crimea, *The International Nursing Review*, in October 1954, reprinted the first Oration in her honor that had previously been delivered at an International Council of Nursing Congress in London during 1937. Entitled "The Commemoration of Florence Nightingale", the article emphasized that she had her faults and made many mistakes. But, in the process, Newman presented an analytical study of her main principles on the way to recognizing Miss Nightingale not only as "the founder of trained nursing but also as one of the international pioneers of the whole science and art of Preventive State Medicine." Since Strachey's *Eminent Victorians* was re-issued in 1948, this reprinting could well be seen as part of the renewed effort at responding to Strachey's iconoclastic portrait.

SIR GEORGE NEWMAN

Florence Nightingale: Pioneer of Preventive State Medicine

It is not without significance that this great representative assembly of nurses of many nations and kindreds and tongues and religions should have one common bond in the great and incomparable name of Miss Florence Nightingale. More than others, you are her soldiers to-day. The life of your illustrious leader, which became a tradition, even a legend, in her own lifetime, is now the treasured possession of the human family all over the world. We do well to remember her here to-day, and count up the thoughts and deeds with which she moved the heart of England. She was born in Florence on May 12th in 1820, and death came to her in London on August 13th, 1910, at the great age of ninety years. Reared as a lady of rank, surrounded by luxury, she lived down the discouragements, and even opposition of her family, and became a hospital nurse, the courageous defender of the sick, the oppressed, "the bad" and the outcast. Though a recluse and for forty years in retirement; what she called "out of office"; she became an eminent public servant of the State. She sought for light in the dark hospital wards at Scutari in 1855, as upon her own lonely path in earlier years, and, finding it, she became to all the world "a lady with a lamp." Longfellow chose her title to fame from the little oil lamp she carried in her hand—"A lady with a lamp I see"—not knowing how true and enduring would prove his choice. In the perplexities of her home life and doubting heart, in the Crimean War, in hospital management, in modern nursing, in sanitary reform, in the emancipation of womanhood, she has proved indeed to be for all time a Lady with a Lamp.

Florence Nightingale's life may be thought of in three subdivisions. First, there is her romantic girlhood and early training, discipline and experience at Kaiserswerth and elsewhere, culminating in what she believed and declared to be "a divine call" or commission to be a hospital nurse. Then secondly, came the short middle period of service under the British War Office as "Superintendent of the Female Nursing Establishment in the English General Military Hospitals in Turkey" for two years during the Crimean War (1854-56), which created her fame and brought to her the homage of the world. Lastly, there was third period of the remaining forty years of her active life (1856-1895) filled to the brim with an amazing output of constructive statecraft. When we come to consider it carefully, and critically, historically, scientifically and without the aid of the invention of "cunningly devised fables," we find it a most amazing record. Its length, its variety, its adventure, its combination of recluse and publicist, of aristocrat and democrat, of religious mystic and practical reformer; its astounding volume of industry, year in, year out, over three generations; its insight and foresight; its world-wide comprehension, and its tremendous harvest—all contribute to make her life a story standing by itself in the history of mankind.

Surrounding this central figure moves a host of men and women, the most eminent of their day—soldiers, sailors, statesmen, proconsuls, doctors, engineers, poets, theologians, philosophers—thwarting or abetting her, obeying or refusing her bidding, rejected or inspired by her. They pass before us like ghosts out of the long past. They come and go, they live and labour and die around this remarkable woman, who seems to go marching on to her special destiny, undeviating, undefeated, undismayed, lord of her own event. Sometimes she is like a Hebrew prophet, warning, foretelling, declaiming and declaring; sometimes as practical mystic, like her friends, Sidney Herbert, Lord Lawrence of the Punjab, and General Gordon; sometimes as reformer like Lord Shaftesbury; Miltonic in austerity, of intensive fire like Savonarola or Francis of Assisi; a theologian like Dean Stanley or Professor Jowett; an adult educationalist, a scientific investigator with Dr. Parkes and Dr. Farr; a philosopher like her friend John Stuart Mill; an artist in taste after the school of Giotto in the fourteenth century; a soldier in understanding and command, *and all the time a hospital nurse*—always observing and collating, always for bold action, always ready and reliable when needed, sometimes to be persuaded, sometimes immovable as a rock—"as the shadow of a great rock in a weary land."

We all know, in a general way, what Miss Nightingale did for the wounded of three nations in the Crimean War. As Kinglake, the historian, said: "There acceded to the State a new power," and Professor Trevelyan has added his considered opinion in these words:

> The real hero of the War was Florence Nightingale, and its indubitable outcome was modern nursing, both military and civil, a new conception of the potentiality and place in society of the trained and educated woman, and a juster national conception of the character and claims of the private soldier.

There is something for us to think about. What Miss Nightingale did in the Crimean War was to open widely the gates of order and efficiency in place of disorder and neglect. She put an end to the tortuous ramifications of administrative incapacity and divided responsibility in the military hospitals; an end to the inherent faults of confused systems; an end to the scientific ignorance and incompetence of red tape officialism—for these were the three agencies which imperilled the efficiency and health of armies by lending to complacent acquiescence in a high mortality from wounds, and a still higher mortality from preventable disease and starvation. It is strange to reflect upon the fact that this particular problem of excessive mortality among soldiers from disease, though relieved in the Crimean War, did not find its solution until nearly sixty years afterwards in the Great War (1914-1918), with its new knowledge and reformed medical services.

In 1856, after her two dramatic years in the Crimean War, Miss Nightingale, though retired and invalided, turned her genius—alert, determined, apprehending, still purposive—to the wider questions which directly emerged from her experience. Her long years of seclusion were partly due to her physical invalidity, but partly self-designed in order that the serious work of her life might not be hindered by what she considered "the wasted time of claims." Thus only, as she conceived, was she able to carry through her big schemes. It is only possible on this occasion to mention, in order, their main outline.

First, there was the hygiene of the British Army, and Miss Nightingale's initiation of, and work for, the Royal Commission on the health of the Army in 1857, concurrently with which there was issued her "Notes affecting the health, efficiency and hospital administration of the British Army." Her conception of the health of the soldier included his social welfare, his character, his training, his food and sleep, his cleanliness, his leisure, his savings, his letters home, his own people. "She was the soldier's friend, no less than the ministering angel."

The Report of the Royal Commission, including a special Memorandum by herself of thirty folio pages, was published in 1858, and was followed by the establishment of the Army Medical School; by reform in hospital construction and the renovation of the military barrack system, and by the improvement in the collection and arrangement of army medical statistics. To Miss Nightingale, the science of medical statistics was almost a religious exercise, a compass, a signpost which she approached with reverence, the ascertainment of the truth of conditions and their effect.

Then came the far-reaching problem of the necessity for the adequate training of nurses, the establishment in 1860 of the Nightingale Training School (provided by Miss Nightingale out of the National Fund presented to herself as a public tribute to her Crimean work), and by its personal direction, the creation of a nursing profession. As a prelude to this great movement, Miss Nightingale had published her popular but classic "Notes on Nursing: What it is and what it is not," in 1859; an epoch-making little book, both of current technique and of enduring wisdom.

The foundation of the training of nurses was followed by her initiation of a Royal Commission on the Sanitary State of the Army in India, which reported in 1863. It is important to remember that such an enquiry had been foreshadowed by her in 1857 at the end of her Notes on the British Army printed in that year and published in 1858. "It would be a noble beginning," she said, "of the new order of things (after the Indian Mutiny) *to use hygiene as the handmaid of civilisation.*" The method she suggested included sanitary commissioners in India under the Government of India but also supervised by the India Office in England, and his being adopted by the Commission was announced in due course by her friend Sir John Lawrence, the Viceroy. It is not surprising that she should say, "I sing for joy every day at John Lawrence's Government." It was indeed a great partnership and it began in fact the reorganisation of the public health service in India on a wide basis, including sanitary commissioners, the sanitation of villages and soldiers' barracks and military stations, land irrigation, hospitals and prisons, and the prevention of periodical famine.

Hardly less pregnant was Miss Nightingale's contribution to the reform of nursing under the Poor Law in England. Miss Twining and Dr. Rogers began such reform in London in 1853. But in 1861, Miss Nightingale co-operated with Mr. William Rathbone of Liverpool in introducing her friend and disciple, Miss Agnes Jones, "a Nightingale probationer" to the workhouse infirmary at Liverpool. The Liverpool experiment of using trained nurses in poor law institutions sealed the doom of the untrained "pauper nurses," though they did not officially disappear for many years. Indeed, two generations had to pass before the Nursing Order of the Local Government Board in 1913 fulfilled Miss Nightingale's first principles of Poor Law nursing, and it was not until Mr. Neville Chamberlain's great Local Government Act of 1929 (which itself incorporated several of the chief principles enunciated by Miss Nightingale in 1886) that the crucial victory was really won. Thus she introduced the special training and wider sphere of nurses, midwives and health visitors.

Lastly, there was the supreme principle of the "neutralisation" of the wounded soldier, of whatever nationality. Somewhere about 1743 Sir John Pringle, the British founder of modern military medicine, suggested that military hospitals should be regarded as neutral and immune from attack by any of the fighting forces. This far-reaching rule remained without national or international support until the experience of the Crimean War of 1854 and the Italian War of 1859 moved Henri Dunant, Swiss philanthropist (himself inspired by Miss Nightingale's work at Scutari) to describe the barbarities of war and in particular the necessity of protecting the wounded. He instigated the consideration of this principle at the Geneva "Society of Public Service" in February, 1863, and subsequently secured direct attention to it at two international conferences convoked at Geneva in 1863 and 1864. In August of the latter year was instituted the international "Geneva Convention" which formulated the principle of the neutralisation of the wounded under the Red Cross, and it was Miss Nightingale herself who, at the request of the British War Office, drafted the instructions for the British delegates at that Convention, to support the declaration of the neutrality of Red Cross Hospitals, doctors, nurses, and all wounded soldiers. It was but expressing in definite compendious terms her practice in the Crimea of nursing all wounded men of whatever nationality, friend or foe.

Here then we have our Lady's programme of public service. What are we to make of her and of it? First, respecting herself we may discard all legendary fancies, fables, fabrications, and the inflated and uncertain atmosphere of "romance," and, if we can, we must weigh as in a balance the actual facts which remain after seventy years of opinion, and of praise or blame or misinterpretation. Miss Nightingale's character was, like all human character, a complex of heredity and environment, but in her case it was the resultant also of the use of high spiritual forces and will-power in varied circumstance. She was able to prearrange much of the circumstances of her life (as in large measure we can all do), and considered it to be her duty to do so, in order to make both her life and her nursing work directly conducive to what she conceived to be her mission. Moreover, she took pains to develop a capacity and an insight to capture from circumstance its *elements of guidance*, and in this sense could justly have preferred the ancient claim *"I control circumstance, not circumstance me?"* It has been said that she was paradoxical, vacillating, opinionated, autocratic, intolerant, prejudiced, self-willed, masterful, and in discipline even a martinet. Well, ninety years is a very long period of life, and I daresay that on occasion Miss Nightingale manifested, like the rest of us, each of these qualities. They do not disturb me in the least; they are human, common to us all, and in any army leader sometimes unavoidable. Quite naturally and properly she was nicknamed "The Bird," and it is curious to note how its varied plumage appeared to different observers; a swallow, a martin, a duckling, a dove, a nightingale, a swan, or an eagle; it is perilous at this date to specify. Perhaps from time to time she had some of the characteristics of all these beautiful birds, certainly of the last named!

Ruskin told us that in order to judge works of consummate Art, it is necessary to give them both *time* and *space*. And in truth we must stand off some distance to measure or differentiate this great and preeminent person—for great and entirely exceptional, history will assuredly declare her to be. This at least may be said, the plain facts show that she was a woman of sound and practical common sense, compassionate and tender-hearted, diligent, loyal, *self-renouncing because self-dedicated*, with a genius for administrative organisation, possessing a high sense of public duty and statesmanship, and with a soul anchored in the inexhaustible and enduring verities of her religious faith and her spiritual experience—still the greatest power on earth to move the minds and hearts of men and women.

We must not assume that in Miss Nightingale we have unapproachable impeccability, some kind of hypothetical sinlessness and perfection. No. she had her faults and no doubt made many mistakes, for she was constituted of the same clay as ourselves. She belonged to an age different from our own, the nineteenth and not the twentieth century. She was surrounded for two whole generations by criticism and controversy, some of it self-created, and we must not be rash or impatient in our ultimate estimates. Indeed not the least of her personal achievements was that, like an alchemist, she *transmuted* in the course of years the nature, form and substance of the conventionalities of her own social environment and its standards and judgments, changing them from baser metal into gold. Let me recall to your remembrance Lord Rosebery's appraisement of the deductions and allowances which we must make for human nature, one of the most beautiful passages in modern English:

> When we see that the greatest and choicest images of God have had their weaknesses like ours. their temptations, their hours of darkness, their bloody sweat; are we not encouraged by their lapses and catastrophes to find energy for one more effort, one more struggle? Where they failed, we feel it a less dishonour to fail; their errors and sorrows make, as it were, an easier ascent from infinite imperfection to infinite perfection.
>
> Man, after all, is not ripened by virtue alone. Were it so, this world were a paradise of angels. No, like the growth of the earth, he is the fruit of all the seasons; the accident of a thousand accidents, a living mystery, moving through the seen to the unseen. He is sown in dishonour; he is matured under all the varieties of heat and cold; in mist and wrath, in snow and vapours, in the melancholy of autumn, in the topor of winter, as well as in the rapture and fragrance of summer, or the balmy affluence of the spring—its breath, its sunshine, its dew. And at the end he is reaped—the product not of one climate, but of all; not of good alone, but of evil; not of joy alone, but of sorrow—perhaps mellowed and ripened, perhaps stricken, and withered and sour. How then shall we judge anyone? How at any rate shall we judge a giant, great in gifts and great in temptation, great in strength and great in weakness? Let us glory in his strength and be comforted in his weakness.

Finally, I turn to say a word of summary upon Miss Nightingale's workmanship. It was varied and prolonged, yet it was all of one piece, with little or no alien element or diversion from a straight line of purpose. An analytical study of her main principles, as interpreted in her practices, suggests that, speaking generally, they were six in number:

(a) The national and social importance of the hygiene of armies, and to that end the hygiene also of *the classes of society from which the soldier is drawn*;

(b) *The* necessity of adopting the principles of science and art in designing hospital construction and management, and in the improvement of national sanitation;

(c) The more accurate and fuller recording of the incidence and definition of disease, sickness and incapacity, physical and mental; in order to discover the foundation both of truth and of action;

(d) The absolute requirement of adequate training for nurses, midwives and health workers, if they are to prove efficient and worth while, and *the application of their beneficent services to all classes of the community;*

(e) The emancipation and education of the womanhood of a nation to be approximately equivalent to that of its manhood;

(f) A universal law for the international neutralisation of the wounded soldier, as the *irreducible minimum of civilisation* as against barbarism.

No one can read this formidable list without recognising that Miss Nightingale was not only the founder of trained nursing, she was also one of the international pioneers of the whole science and art of Preventive State Medicine, which is today so profoundly affecting, transforming and expanding man's life upon the earth. It should, however, be observed that, though she was concerned in each of these six enterprises, she wove them together like a single piece of tapestry, a synthetic philosophy. Yet she did not finish or complete any one of them. They are still incomplete, and in each sphere there remains much to do. In order that her disciples may make their contribution, they will bear in mind that, though they may wisely endeavour to emulate, they should not attempt to imitate Miss Nightingale. We may appreciate her as a national and international possession for which the human family must ever be grateful, but we shall not heighten or enhance such appreciation by allowing "the dead hand of the past" to be laid too heavily upon us. She herself would have said that advance in *new times, new knowledge* and *new methods* is still greatly needed in all six directions, though not equally needed in all nations. We are not called upon to pledge ourselves today that we also will *do* what Miss Nightingale *did*—it cannot be—but we may fairly aspire, in our own problems and in our own lands, times and ways, to act upon the high plane of her motive and objectives, expanding both their occasion and operation.

In the presence of an international assembly of nurses for the healing of the nations, one can hardly escape the reflection, what an inestimable gain for the whole world it would be if, as well as neutralising the wounded men and women of our generation, each nation would learn the wisdom of neutralising its traditional lack of appreciation of other nations, the mutual undervaluations and particular shortcomings, and the ignorance and prejudices which so easily beset us all.

For, to *know* and *understand* is always to make juster judgments of men. Our true valuation of Florence Nightingale would find most appropriate expression, yes, and would choose the better part; first, in gratefully accepting with knowledge and with understanding, the inspiration of her life and work and its spiritual foundation; and secondly, in planning our own day's enterprise in order that it shall both *extend the frontiers* and *enlarge* its opportunity for the men, women and children of all nations.''

Previous selections in this section have examined, in particular, her post-Crimean successes as author, reformer and pioneer. This article, written on the 150th anniversary of her birth, is a clear effort by one of the leading American nursing journals to publicize Florence Nightingale's legacy to nursing. Authored by the journal's Senior Associate Editor, the article asked, for example: "How can one woman accomplish all that she did?" The answer provided was blatantly and deliberately un-Strachey-like: "Miss Nightingale's deeply religious convictions that found their outlet in works of benefit to humanity. She chose to live a life that was meaningful to her." Moreover, in anticipation of the final section to follow, Isler poignantly reminds her fellow nurses that Florence Nightingale's legacy to nursing— "of knowledge, humanitarianism, and compassion—is timeless."

CHARLOTTE ISLER

"Florence Nightingale: Rebel with a Cause"

In 1970, every hospital worthy of the name provides clean beds, sanitary surroundings, proper nutrition, and a well-qualified staff of physicians and nurses capable of giving quality patient care.

Consider the situation 150 years ago. The Industrial Revolution was already well under way in Europe and the United States, but conditions in hospitals of that period were so deplorable that only a major revolution could change them. That such a revolution took place is now history. That it was largely brought about through the efforts of one woman is little short of a miracle.

The hospitals of that day were dumping places for the poor. Surgery (mostly amputations) combined risk with torture, for anesthesia was not yet in use. Sanitation was unknown, and patients were seldom bathed or the bed linens changed. Infections often killed more patients than did the diseases that had brought the patients to the hospital. Custodial care was given by women who were paupers, drunkards, or prostitutes, unfit for any other work. Many of them were forced to work in hospitals for punitive reasons, with the result that they victimized rather than cared for their charges.

Into this social milieu, came Florence Nightingale, an English gentlewoman. To understand how courageous her action was, one must consider "woman's place" in that day. The daughters of respectable families never entered the working world. A wealthy wife might bestow charity by taking food to the poor and sick, or giving money. But no respectable woman ever nursed the poor, as much because she didn't know what to do as because it wouldn't have been proper.

Miss Nightingale lifted herself above society's restriction. To the hospital she brought sanitation, reforms in construction, and systematic and increasingly skilled nursing care. Under her influence, nursing developed into a complex profession, and hospitals became places where people went to get well, not to die.

How could one woman accomplish all this? The answer lies in Miss Nightingale's deeply religious convictions that found their outlet in works of benefit to humanity. She chose to live a life that was meaningful to her.

THE EARLY YEARS

Florence Nightingale was born on May 12, 1820, while her family was in Florence, Italy, Her parents were well-to-do and well educated, and she had one older sister, Parthenope. The girls were privileged to grow up in a beautiful English country home, where they led a happy and protected life.

Florence had the good luck to have a highly intelligent, perceptive father who noticed quite early that she showed exceptional intelligence. He tutored her himself in mathematics, languages, religion, and philosophy. As she grew older, study whetted her appetite for more knowledge. This was a great satisfaction to her father; but her mother felt that Florence, who was growing into a beautiful and clever young lady, would do better to display more interest in the household arts.

By the time she was 17, Florence was discontented with her life. She and her sister, Parthe, had been presented at Queen Victoria's court. Though Florence was now an accomplished dancer and a brilliant conversationalist, she began to show an aversion to the endless round of social events that occupied the family. Even the flattering attentions of the many young men who courted her—making Parthe quite jealous of her more popular sister—couldn't change the feeling she had that she should be living a more useful life.

That year (1837) she made the following entry in her diary: "God spoke to me and called me to His service."

At first she had no idea how she could serve. But through conversations with some of her philanthropic friends, she learned of the misery of the sick poor, and particularly the hospital inmates. Then she learned from the Prussian ambassador, a family friend, about a Pastor Fliedner of Kaiserswerth, Germany, who had established a 100-bed hospital run by deaconesses. Her conviction grew that hospital work was her calling.

Florence immediately began studying all the information she could find about hospitals. But when she told her partents of her plans, they objected violently. (Parthe had hysterics.) It would, they felt, ruin the family reputation if they let her have her way.

With characteristic determination, Florence secretly continued her preparation. She persuaded sympathetic friends to supply her with charts, reports, and other documents concerning hospitals all over Europe, and she studied them when alone at night. In 1847, when she was 27, she spoke to the American philanthropist Dr. Ward Howe, asking his opinion of her plan "to devote myself to works of charity in hospitals." He urged her to go ahead if she felt this was her vocation. She enlisted the aid of a family friend, the chief physician of a nearby hospital, who agreed to let her learn nursing under his supervision.

Her parents' answer was still an unqualified No.

Nervous symptoms resulted from her frustration and enforced idleness; she became severely depressed and took to her bed. Several proposals of marriage had added to her psychological burden. She had fallen deeply in love several times, but had rejected each suitor because she felt she could not combine her "vocation," as she interpreted it, with marriage and family responsibility. To distract her, friends took her abroad. In each city, she visited hospitals and took volumes of notes for study and comparison.

Finally, in 1851, when she was 31, her parents grudgingly gave her permission to go to Kaiserswerth and work under Pastor Fliedner and his wife. There she found the compassionate attitude that was so sorely lacking in other hospitals she had visited. She stayed three months. During that time she came to realize the importance of systematic nursing based on knowledge of the body, its diseases, and how to treat them; and she found that not even Kaiserswerth provided this kind of nursing. At last she knew what it was she was meant to do: put her years of study and observation to work to improve the quality of hospitals and of nursing care.

Her first opportunity came in 1853, when she was offered the position of superintendent of the Institution for Sick Gentlewomen in Distressed Circumstances, a hospital being set up in London to care for governesses and other ladies. Her father, at last receptive to her wishes, gave her a yearly allowance (never forgiven by her mother). She received no salary, and even had to pay the salary of the house-keeper who came with her to "insure her respectability."

After supervising all preparations in the building on Harley Street, Florence quickly proved to the medical and lay boards of the institution that she was an expert at innovation as well as administration. First she concentrated on staff discipline. Sobriety was essential, and so was appropriate behavior while on duty. Any nurses, cooks, other employees, and even doctors who did not meet these requirements were asked to leave.

Many of her suggestions startled and upset the conservative board, but she gained her points one by one: A lift was built to carry patients' food to the upper floors (and save weary nurses' legs). Call bells were installed, and hot water was piped to each floor. Clean linen was provided for each patient—and even more miraculous—changed at regular intervals. Food was prepared and cooked in accordance with Florence's studies on nutrition. She insisted on admitting patients on a nonsectarian basis.

Her patients adored her. She was kind and considerate, and often helped them with funds out of her own pocket. She taught her nurses what she had learned, and for the first time in her life felt completely happy. She continued her habit of observing and taking notes. Progress, she knew, could only come from hard facts, the prerequisites for further improvements.

THE CALL TO WAR

Less than a year after Florence had assumed her post at Harley Street, she was offered a more important post at London's Kings College Hospital. But she never accepted, for an even greater challenge had arisen.

The year before (1853), the Crimean War between Russia on the one side and Britain, Turkey, and France had broken out. Now frightening reports were reaching England from the war correspondent for The Times of London. Due to lack of planning, negligence, and incredible mismanagement, many British troops lacked even such essentials as food and warm clothing. Cholera, typhoid, and other disease had broken out, and the death rate was soaring. Troops got sick and died without ever seeing the enemy.

Medical provisions, supplies, and equipment were unobtainable—even beds and mattresses. The wounded had to be transported from the front lines in the Crimea across the stormy Black Sea to a base hospital in Scutari, Turkey, on the outskirts of Constantinople (now Istanbul). Men were dying like flies from exposure, starvation, and lack of medical and nursing care.

Florence had become Britain's foremost authority on hospitals and nursing. She knew that her youth and her sex were against her, but she felt she must offer her services to relieve the suffering of the troops. She volunteered in a formal letter to Sir Sidney Herbert, Secretary for War and a personal friend. At the very same time, Sir Sidney—embarrassed by the shocking disclosures and deeply concerned—sent a formal note to Florence requesting her to head an official mission. Her assignment: to go to Scutari in charge of a party of nurses and perform, under the supervision of the chief medical officer, whatever nursing services she deemed necessary.

Florence accepted at once. Within five days she had recruited 38 nurses. Before departing to undertake her difficult and dangerous task, she received a letter from her mother wishing her well, and another from the man who had meant more to her than any other suitor. Referring to the war, he wrote her in one of his letters: "You can undertake THAT when you could not undertake me!"

Florence and her nurses had expected problems, but the hardships they met in Scutari went beyond anything they could have foreseen. It was clear that the military authorities were far from enthusiastic about having a group of "meddlesome females" among them.

The nurses were shown to a dingy little suite of rooms in one of the towers of the enormous barracks hospital, totally inadequate for 39 women. A dead Turkish Army officer was sprawled grotesquely across one of the beds. Filth and vermin were everywhere. When Florence made her first modest requests for scrubbing brushes, bedding, clothing, and other essentials, her requisitions were held up by red tape or conflicting regulations, or were returned because of "empty stores." Her task seemed insuperable. ("There should be a sign," she noted grimly in a letter home: "Abandon Hope All Ye Who Enter Here.")

But Florence had come prepared for shortages. During the journey from England, she had bought supplies she thought might be needed; using funds contributed to her group at home. Whatever the Army stores wouldn't or couldn't provide, she did. Two close friends, Mr. and Mrs. Bracebridge, had come to Scutari with her. Now she put them to work as purchasing agents, searching the shops of Constantinople for what was needed. Meanwhile, she co-operated to the best of her ability with the military and medical authorities despite their opposition.

Acceptance came soon. Two disastrous battles (Balaclava and Inkerman) sent hundreds of wounded and dying soldiers to Scutari, swamping the facilities. To complicate matters, an expected supply ship was sunk en route by a hurricane. Suddenly the goodwill Florence had shown, the help provided by her hardworking nurses, and particularly the desperately needed supplies she had furnished from her own resources finally won the cooperation of the medical officers.

In turn, Florence insisted that her nurses cooperate with them. Nurses were required to have an order signed by a doctor before carrying out treatment. They were to be available to help the doctors in all procedures where needed. Any nurse who was promiscuous or found drunk was unceremoniously sacked and shipped home. Florence's discipline did not suit all her nurses, and disagreements occurred. Also, friction with a number of senior medical officers continued, notably with Sir John Hall, chief medical officer in the Crimea. For Florence did not hesitate to brand as stupid, inefficient, or reprehensible such actions as seemed to merit such descriptions, and she sent many critical letters to the War Office.

Despite continuing strife, Florence and her nurses made enormous progress. By summer, 1855, there were 125 nurses under her command. The troops brought to the hospital found clean beds and clothes, nourishing food, and special diet (Florence had engaged a French culinary expert), and all received treatment and medications.

The men idolized her. She made it a point to stay with them in their worst hours—during surgery to remove bullets or amputations, for example, usually done without anesthesia. On rounds, she took notes, listened to requests, and made improvements. In less than a year's time, improvements in patient care reduced the death rate from a staggering 42 per 100 to a low of 22 per 1,000.

During 1855 she had a serious bout with "Crimean Fever" that left her weak and with permanent effects. Yet her concern for the troops continued. She saw there was no place for the convalescent men to stay, and drunkenness was a major problem. "Give them something worthwhile to do," she reasoned, "and they'll drink less and start sending home some of their pay."

Despite the officers' indifference and scepticism, Florence insisted on setting up a recreation room (the Inkerman Café) where coffee, books, magazines, and writing materials were available. She also arranged for a more reliable system for soldiers to use to send their pay home.

Within a short time, thousands of pounds (British currency) were being sent home to families on a regular basis, proving the soundness of her belief in rehabilitation and in the good character of the much-maligned British soldier.

The war ended in April, 1856. Florence stayed at Scutari until after the last soldier had been discharged from the hospital. All the way home she was haunted by the memory of the dead—not only those killed in battle but also the 9,000 that had died of disease in just six months. Back in England she was hailed as a national heroine to be honored and feted, and her family hoped that, now that the war was over, she would return to the old way of life.

Both the nation and her family were disappointed. For she avoided all celebrations, and she refused to return to her family. She had proved the value of female nurses to the military and to her country. But she could not forget the soldiers who had died because of ignorance, neglect, and preventable diseases. She was determined to bring about reforms in barracks construction, military sanitation, and the Army's medical department.

While at Scutari, she had met members of various Government commissions sent there (often at her request) to investigate the military hospitals, barracks, medical and other equipment or lack of it. These men, aghast at what they had found, now collaborated with her and with influential men such as Sir Sidney Herbert to effect reforms. A new peacetime commission had to be authorized with power to make needed changes. This was a touchy political issue, and findings were likely to embarrass many officials.

Florence was summoned to appear before Queen Victoria. She put her case before the queen so effectively that Victoria immediately requested action on forming such a commission. She was so impressed by Florence's presentation of her views that she wrote to her commander-in-chief: "I wish we had HER at the War Office."

Once the commission started its work, the members had to rely almost exclusively on Florence's notes, observations, and documents as evidence. She could not be a member of the commission herself because she was a woman, but in effect she was its most active member. Though ill and weak much of the time, and pestered by her mother and sister who had joined her in her London hotel to attend the social season, she put in endless hours preparing a lengthy book on her experiences and findings during the war*. Simultaneously, she wrote

---

*Title: "Notes on Matters Affecting the Health, Efficiency, and Hospital Administration of the British Army: Founded Chiefly on the Experience of the Late War."

a detailed report, presented subsequently to the new Secretary for War, Lord Panmure.

As a result of her work, an amazing number of reforms were undertaken. Female Army nursing was firmly established. Nutrition was improved for the soldiers. Barracks and hospital construction and regulations were changed and improved. An Army medical school was established. (Florence had reported that young Army doctors were woefully lacking in a knowledge of military medicine). Special medical instruction was given to selected soldiers, who thus became the first "corpsmen" trained to give skilled care to the sick and wounded.

Florence was especially eager to have the barracks reforms instituted quickly, for she had found that even in peacetime the mortality rate of soldiers in Army barracks was double or more than double that of civilians living in the same area. "Our soldiers enlist to death in the barracks" was her slogan that helped push through the suggested improvements.

The strain of long working hours, fear of failure, and her mother's and sister's inconsiderate behavior took their toll during these years. Several times Florence felt so bitter, ill, and exhausted that she made her will, certain she did not have long to live. But each time she rallied, and forced herself to continue her projects.

Her reputation had now grown to such dimensions that she was in continual demand as a consultant. Authorities abroad as well as at home sought her opinion before they built new hospitals or made decisions regarding military medicine and nursing. In the United States, Civil War nurse Dorothea Dix, among others, received her counsel in 1861 when Miss Dix was appointed superintendent of nurses in Washington.

THE GREAT EXPERIMENT

It had become clear to Florence that nursing care as she envisioned it would never be a reality unless and until a systematic way of training well-qualified nurses could be developed. Fortunately, she had the means at hand to undertake the first serious experiment in nursing education: a large sum of money given by the public in 1855 to honor her contribution to the war.

Arrangements were made to establish the Nightingale Training School at old St. Thomas' Hospital, London, under a one-year contract. Mrs. Wardroper, the hospital superintendent, was the first matron. Florence planned the school's 12-month program and personally interviewed each prospective probationer. On June 24, 1860, the historic first class of 15 probationers entered training.

Florence was determined to prove that by carefully selecting young women (ages 25-35) and giving them good training and spiritual and moral guidance, nursing could be raised from its low reputation to a respectable and even prestigious profession. She personally supervised each detail of the program: ward teaching, lectures, design of the students' living quarters, their indoor and outdoor uniforms, even their recreation activities. She discussed with Mrs. Wardroper every new development, however trivial. She wrote the probationers letters of encouragement, and urged them to confide in her if they had problems. She also devised report forms, then checked and evaluated the performance reports written by the matron.

Her comments were always succinct, if not always flattering: "Nurse E. gets up early to misinform herself; terrible gossip, flighty, flirty, not thorough, no use." Or, "If there is anything in her, it requires a hand pump to get it out."

She was equally interested in the instructors' performances, as evaluated by her and as revealed in students' reports and assigned diaries. ("Sister A. taught me nothing," wrote one student.) Florence herself had stated: "Theory without practice is ruinous to nurses." Now she came to see that the reverse was also true.

What had begun as a one-year experiment became an immediate success. In 1871 St. Thomas' Hospital moved into new quarters, making it possible to further improve the nurses' training program. Lectures by doctors and nurses were steadily expanded. Eventually a preliminary seven-week training course was added, and a full-time "sister tutor" (instructor of nursing) was employed.

With success came a great cry for "Nightingales," as the school's graduates were called. The Nightingale Fund Council, administrative body of the school, took as much interest in its graduates as it did in its probationers. When a request for a graduate came in, the council made sure the requesting hospital met specified standards or the request would be denied. The hospital had to provide cheerful, well-appointed living quarters for the nurse, a suitable salary, and guarantees that she would be permitted to perform good nursing care. "Nightingales" were often sent out by twos or in larger groups, for mutual support and to better be able to accomplish the invariably necessary reforms.

Florence kept in close touch with the graduates, as volumes of her correspondence show. One by one these well-trained, dedicated women turned her vision of nursing as an art and a profession into fact. "Nightingales" brought skilled nursing care to the sick poor in hospitals, in workhouse infirmaries, and finally, at Florence's instigation, into their homes as well. For she was farsighted enough to see the need for "district nursing" (public health nursing).

Countries such as Australia, France, and the United States pleaded for Nightingale graduates or asked for help in setting up nursing schools on the Nightingale Plan. One of the earliest graduates, Lucy Osburn (class of 1867), and five other nurses went to Sydney, Australia. Another early graduate, Alice Fisher (class of 1875), established several nursing schools in Britain and then sailed to America in 1884 to establish a school at Philadelphia's 3,000-bed Blockley Hospital. Other U.S. hospitals that set up schools on the Nightingale Plan included Bellevue, 1873; University of Pennsylvania, 1886; and Johns Hopkins, 1889.

The Nightingale Training School continued to grow in size and international reputation. By 1887 more than 500 nurses had been graduated, and they were upgrading hospitals and nursing all over the world.

Florence, meanwhile, had been occupied with many projects. Her sister had finally married, and her father had bought Florence a house in London, providing the freedom she had so long wanted. In 1859 she had published her famous "Notes on Nursing," an immediate best seller. "Notes on Hospitals" had come out in 1863, followed later by other equally important works.

An excellent writer, Florence documented her observations with clarity and wit. In her introduction to "Hospitals," for instance, she states: "It may seem a strange principle to enunciate as the very first requirement in a hospital that it should do the sick no harm."

Throughout these years, Florence was a partial invalid. The palpitations, nausea at the sight of food, and insomnia she suffered were partly a leftover from the hardships of the Crimean War, perhaps, and partly a reaction to family pressures and other intrusions into her personal life. She rarely went out, hardly ever attended public functions, saw people only by appointment and then only one at a time. She spent most of her days on a couch, working on books, research papers, or correspondence. Being a partial invalid freed her to make full use of her creative capacities. She drove herself just as she drove others who worked with her, and often wrote day and night until a project was completed.

The nurse mortality rate—much higher in that day than that of other women of comparable ages—was a subject of burning interest to Florence. "The loss of a well-trained nurse by preventable disease," she wrote, "is a greater loss than is that of a good soldier from the same cause. Money cannot replace either, but a good nurse is more difficult to find than a good soldier."

Of equally great interest to her was the maternal mortality rate, which was shockingly high in Britain and even worse abroad. With characteristic precision, she made use of statistics in trying to determine its causes—another "first" in nursing and medicine. Questionnaires she devised and sent to hospitals at home and abroad revealed a maternal death rate due to childbirth of up to 33 deaths per 1,000 births in Britain, up to 95 deaths per 1,000 elsewhere in Europe.

She discovered that the death rate was invariably lowest among women who delivered at home, no matter how poor or ill-kept the home was. The death rate soared in hospitals where women were crowded into small rooms, or stayed for any length of time, or were cared for by doctors and nurses who also cared for other types of patients. (Women in lying-in hospitals, where no other patients were admitted, did much better.) The worst death rate by far was that of the teaching hospitals where medical students were allowed to examine parturient women as well as other patients, and also perform autopsies.

Asepsis and antisepsis were still years away, and even Semmelweis's handwashing theory was unknown outside Vienna. The recommendations Florence made, based on her statistical research, in "Introductory Notes on Lying-In Institutions" (1871) saved thousands of mothers.

THE FINAL YEARS

Florence Nightingale lived to see nursing develop to the point where its leaders began looking toward professional organization and official recognition of the profession through certification by the government. She opposed certification(licensure) because it meant each nurse must pass a standard examination, and she felt that the "art of nursing" could not be standardized in this way. (In England, state licensure became a reality nine years after her death.)

In her last years Florence continued to take an active interest in nursing. After her father and mother died, she spent much time at Claydon House, her sister Parthe's home. The 89-year-old Sir Harry Verney, Bart., D.S.O. (grandson of Parthe and her husband, Sir Harry Verney), remembers this period of Florence's life with great affection. She was his favorite great aunt, who understood children better than any other adult. In a recent conversation at the Verney family estate in Buckinghamshire, England, he told of her kindness, her cheerfulness, her unfailing understanding of and generosity towards children. Too old to care for patients, she transferred all her affection to the children who came to her with their problems, confident that she would know how to solve them.

The kindly old woman whose iron determination to make nursing a skilled profession had left its mark on nursing everywhere died on August 13, 1910. She had been showered with honors towards the end of her life, but she had cared little for those. It was the work itself and the achievement that had mattered to her. To make the profession of nursing into what she knew it could become, she had been willing to spend much of her life in seclusion.

Now, on the 150th anniversary of her birth, what can be said of her legacy to nursing?

Nursing today is an acknowledged profession all over the world, and nursing services play an indispensable role in every health-care system and specialty. Nursing education has expanded continuously to keep pace with medical advances, in the Nightingale tradition. The Florence Nightingale Education Division of the International Council of Nurses, the National Memorial Committee (of Great Britain and Ireland), The Florence Nightingale Memorial Fund in Britain, and a similar fund just launched in Baltimore, Md., continue to honor her name by providing grants and scholarships for advanced study by nurses.

More than 100 years ago Florence Nightingale expounded the philosophy of flexibility that still guides nursing today: "Everything which succeeds is not the production of a scheme (plan), or rules and regulations made beforehand, but of a mind observing and adapting itself to wants and events." Her words still ring true in the Space Age. Her legacy to nursing—of knowledge, humanitarianism, and compassion —is timeless.

Florence Nightingale and the Birth of Professional Nursing

William J. Bishop was the editor of *Medical History* and original editor of *A Bio-Bibliography of Florence Nightingale* prior to his untimely death in July, 1961. Bishop, a librarian and medical historian, spent the last seven years of his life in an intensive study and accumulation of the published writings of Florence Nightingale in preparation for compiling a catalogue of her correspondence. This project, initiated and supported by the International Council of Nurses (ICN) and the Florence Nightingale International Foundation (FNIF), was later completed by his assistant and secretary Sue Goldie and published in 1962. The article selected for this section was based on an address delivered by Bishop at the 1959 National League of Nursing Convention in Philadelphia. Serving as a preview to the later *Bio-Bibliography,* the emphasis is on how "it is in her letters that she unbares her soul and expresses her inmost thoughts; it was through her letters that she planned and plotted and bent people to her will." Through this study of her vast correspondence, according to Bishop, "the prevision of this extraordinary woman was such that it has taken the world a hundred years to catch up with some of her ideas and principles."

WILLIAM J. BISHOP

"Florence Nightingale's Message for Today"

The vast correspondence carried on by Florence Nightingale throughout her long, rich, and busy life provides a unique key to what this great woman thought and what she accomplished—ideas and achievements which far transcend her work for nursing, great though that was. Her interests had enormous breadth and scope, and we are fortunate indeed to have her letters to show us so much of the person she really was.

Miss Nightingale's most important written work appeared in the form of the reports of governmental commissions—huge volumes replete with minutes of evidence and masses of statistics, yet even these volumes contain many flashes of wit and humor. But it is in her letters that we find the characteristic sallies, the crushing sarcasm, the delicate irony and other personal touches that reveal her mind and personality so fully. It is in her letters that she unbares her soul and expresses her inmost thoughts; it was through her letters that she planned and plotted and bent people to her will.

But before going further into the Nightingale correspondence, I should like to mention an aspect of her life and work that has received very little attention—her connections with America and with American medicine and nursing.

I must first make reference to the friendship between Florence Nightingale and Dr. Samuel Gridley Howe, because this had a decisive influence on Miss Nightingale's life. The friendship began in 1844 when Dr. Howe and his wife Julia Ward Howe visited the Nightingale family at Embley, their country home in Hampshire. The Howes, who had been married on April 27, 1843, were making a tour of Europe. Florence Nightingale was then a young woman of 24 who had come to realize the futility of the life of most young girls of her social position, and to feel that she was destined to do some work in the world. Her vital interview with Dr. Howe has been described both by Mrs. Howe in her *Reminiscences* and in the life of Dr. Howe by his daughter, Mrs. Laura E. Richards. According to these accounts, Miss Nightingale met Dr. Howe in the garden one morning before breakfast and posed this question:

> Dr. Howe, you have had much experience in the world of philanthropy; you are a medical man and a gentleman; now may I ask you to tell me, upon your word, whether it would be anything unsuitable or unbecoming to a young English woman, if she should devote herself to work of charity in hospitals and elsewhere as the Catholic Sisters do?

To which Dr. Howe replied:

> My dear Miss Florence, it would be unusual, and in England whatever is unusual is apt to be thought unsuitable; but I say to you, go forward, if you have a vocation for that way of life; act up to your aspiration, and you will find that there is never anything unbecoming or unladylike in doing your duty for the good of others. Choose your path, go on with it, wherever it may lead you, and God be with you!

There seems no doubt that this encouraging reply was a decisive factor in Florence Nightingale's choice of a career. A cordial relationship sprang up between the Howes and Miss Nightingale, and Dr. Howe sent her letters of encouragement and counsel. Her letters in return show her wide reading and her interest in world affairs, an interest that had been stimulated by her travels.

Poor Florence had to endure her personal sense of frustration for some years, but in 1851 she was able to make her fateful visit to Kaiserswerth. On June 20, 1852, she wrote to Dr. Howe, "I went for three months to an Institution of Protestant Deaconesses in Germany last year, at Kaiserswerth—perhaps you may know it. I wish the system could be introduced in England where thousands of women have nothing to do and where hospitals are ill nursed by a class of women not fit to be household servants." An ideal of service had begun to kindle with direction and resolve.

After the death of Dr. Howe his widow sent a copy of her brief memoir of him to Miss Nightingale. In thanking Mrs. Howe for this, Florence wrote, "A great duty has been fulfilled in making known his sympathy for every kind of misfortune—his love of helping humanity, his generous and persevering devotion to right—his noble horror of helpless pity—his indomitable faith in progress . . . And how little he thought of reputation! That was the noblest thing of all." This was Florence Nightingale's tribute to a man whom she described as "one of the best and greatest men of our age."

Florence Nightingale made her own great resolve in 1844, but her career as a nurse did not begin until 1854, when she went to the Crimea. We need not describe the horrors of Balaclava and Scutari. At the end of the war her position was unique and her influence unparalleled. As Benjamin Jowett once said to her, "You are a myth in your own lifetime". In establishing that legend, no one played a more important part than the poet Longfellow whose "Santa Filomena" of 1857 carried the story and the lesson of her life to the hearts of millions:

> Lo! In that hour of misery
> A lady with a lamp I see
> Pass through the glimmering gloom,
> And flit from room to room.
> And slow, as in a dream of bliss,
> The speechless sufferer turns to kiss
> Her shadow, as it falls
> Upon the darkening walls.

When the American Civil War broke out, Miss Nightingale's example in the Crimea produced an immediate effect. On October 8, 1861, she wrote to her friend Dr. William Farr, "Did I tell you that I had forwarded to the War Secretary at Washington, upon application, all our War Office forms and reports, statistical and other, taking the occasion to tell them that, as the United States had adopted our

Registrar-General's nomenclature, it would be easier for them to adopt our Army Statistics Forms." The Women's Central Association of Relief, formed in New York in cooperation with other bodies, petitioned the Secretary of War to appoint a sanitary commission, and this was done. Much of Miss Nightingale's Crimean work was reproduced. An account of the work of the U.S. Sanitary Commission, published in 1864, was dedicated to Florence Nightingale. "All that is herein chronicled," said the author, "you have a right to claim as the result of your own work." The secretary of another body, the U.S. Christian Communion, wrote to Miss Nightingale on July 26, 1865, "Your influence and our indebtedness to you can never be known. Only this is true that everywhere throughout our broad country during these years of inventive and earnest benevolence in the constant endeavour to succour and sustain our heroic defenders, the name and work of Florence Nightingale have been an encouragement and inspiration."

In the same year the plans of an emigrant hospital on Wards Island were sent to her. In return she sent engravings of the departure and arrival of the Pilgrim Fathers with the following note: "Presented to the Commissioners of Emigration of New York for the new Emigrant Hospital on Wards Island by Florence Nightingale as a slight sign of her deepest reverence and her warmest sympathy for the noble act by which they have so magnificently provided for—not their own sick, —those of the Old Country."

From this time onward Miss Nightingale's reputation as a sanitarian and as an expert on hospital design brought her requests from all parts of the world for advice on hospital plans. When the Johns Hopkins hospital was about to be built in 1876, her advice was sought by that great man Dr. John Shaw Billings. "Knowing as I do," he wrote, "the great interest you take in such subjects, I shall consider it as a great favour if . . . you will, if your health permits, examine these plans and the two pamphlets which accompany them and let me know what you think of them." She examined the plans thoroughly and forwarded her suggestions to Dr. Billings. In thanking her, Dr. Billings said, "Your remarks shall be laid before the Trustees as soon as I return to America, and I feel quite sure that they will be very greatly interested in and influenced by your criticisms."

But although Dr. Billings had a high opinion of Miss Nightingale as a hospital planner, he was extremely critical of her nursing system, in particular of the idea of "an independent female hierarchy, which will consider from the very commencement that one of its main objects is to be independent of all males, who are to be considered as the natural enemies of the organization."

Linda Richards, the pioneer nurse of the United States, enjoyed the advantage of postgraduate work at St. Thomas' Hospital and of Miss Nightingale's personal interest and encouragement. Another distinguished Nightingale disciple was that remarkable woman, Alice Fisher. In 1884, Miss Fisher, an early graduate of the Nightingale School who had already reformed the nursing service of three important British hospitals, was invited to accept the post of nursing superintendent of Blockley Hospital in Philadelphia, where she carried through a complete reorganization and founded a school of nursing on Nightingale lines.

In 1872, Dr. W. Gill Wylie, who was then a house surgeon at New York's Bellevue Hospital, went to England to study the Nightingale method of nursing and to report on it to the committee who were organizing the Bellevue Training School for Nurses. On September 18, 1872, Miss Nightingale wrote a letter of 13 pages to Dr. Wylie in which she answered questions which he had put to her and gave a characteristic exposition of her views on the scope and organization of nursing, remarkably succinct and to the point:

> Nurses are not "Medical Men." On the contrary, the nurses are there and solely there *to carry out the orders of the medical and surgical staff* including, of course, the whole practice of cleanliness, fresh air, diet, etc. The whole organization of discipline to which the nurses must be subjected is for the sole purpose of enabling the nurses to carry out intelligently and faithfully such orders and such duties as constitute the whole practice of nursing . . . Their whole training is to enable them to understand how best to carry out medical and surgical orders and the reason why it is to be done *this* way and not *that* way.

When she returned from the Crimea, Florence Nightingale's first concern was the health and welfare of the British soldier. "I stand at the altar of the murdered men," she said, "and while I live I fight their cause." This fight involved the complete reorganization of the medical and nursing services of the army. After this came the foundation of the Nightingale school and the organization of adequate training for nurses, midwives, and health workers who were to make their services available to all classes of the community. Another great work which she accomplished was to secure the adoption of regular principles in hospital construction and management. She became the greatest sanitarian of her age.

In each of these spheres her efforts were at first local or national, but her teaching and influence spread so rapidly that she could soon say with John Wesley, "I look upon the world as my parish." What she did for India would have been more than enough to occupy the lives of ten people of lesser vision and stature. Miss Nightingale was one of the first to call for the more accurate and fuller recording of the incidence of disease. "Statistics," she said, "could reform the world." The Red Cross owed its inception to Henri Dunant, but when that great humanitarian read a paper on the movement, in London in 1872, his first words were:

> Though I am known as the founder of the Red Cross and the originator of the Convention of Geneva, it is to an Englishwoman that all the honour of that convention is due. What inspired me to go to Italy during the War of 1859 was the work of Miss Florence Nightingale in the Crimea.

Finally, it would be almost impossible to exaggerate the part which Florence Nightingale played in the emancipation and education of women.

All this great work was accomplished in the 40 years between 1856 and 1895 by an "invalid" who rarely left her room and never appeared in public. How was it done? Because of the enormous prestige which Miss Nightingale enjoyed, she was for a great part of this period virtually a minister of state without portfolio. Her influence was exerted firstly through royal commissions and departments of state. She was mainly responsible for the appointments to the commissions on the army and on Indian affairs and she drew up their terms of reference; furthermore, she frequently supplied the chairmen with a list of questions to be asked, primed many of the witnesses beforehand, drafted the reports, and saw them through the press. One must remember that the radio was then nonexistent and press had not begun to approach its present ubiquitous position. Miss Nightingale had no public relations officer. Many of her ideas were put out in pamphlets which were privately printed in small numbers and sent to her influential friends in the governing class.

These efforts were reinforced by very occasional interviews (strictly rationed as to time), but far more by "confidential" letters to ministers and members of Parliament. These display her extraordinary grasp of detail, her insight into the essentials of any problem, and her brilliant gifts of exposition and persuasion. The same qualities are shown in her letters to her advisers—the permanent government officials, doctors, and matrons who provided her with ammunition. In studying her correspondence one gets an insight into the breadth of her aims, her motives and her methods. Her style of writing is admirably adapted to the correspondent and to the purpose in hand. Her official letters to ministers are models of clear exposition and cogent reasoning, backed up by facts and figures. She resorts on occasion to flattery, cajolery, scolding, or even downright bullying. Her sly humor is often manifested even in her most serious compositions and her mastery of the pungent phrase might be described as "Churchillian."

Most important, she knew what she was talking about. She could blind a professional statistician with figures; she could discuss the drainage of Bombay or the sewers of Calcutta with the leading engineers of the day; she could write out a complete scheme for the construction of a hospital and for the organization of its nursing service. She could (and I cite actual examples taken from her letters) dash off 10 pages of advice on steam boilers, 13 pages on the use of Parian cement for hospital walls, 12 pages on floor polish, and 6 pages on tea-making.

Her correspondents came from all classes of society and they were spread all over the world. In addition to the letters written to people of power and position there are those written to her servants, to the cottagers on the family estates, to tradespeople, to the mothers of private soldiers, and to hundreds of individuals who sought her advice or who came within the orbit of her multifarious interests and schemes.

In spite of her supposed invalidism—and her letters are full of such phrases as "I am a poor and incurable invalid"—for many years of her life she must have spent 12 or even 15 hours a day in writing. Many of her letters were written at 4 or 5 A.M.—"by candlelight," as she is often at pains to note. She frequently wrote to the same person three or four times in the course of one day. A great many letters are marked "confidential" or "private-burn," but these admonitions did not prevent the recipients from preserving the letters with the greatest care. Fortunately, her handwriting is bold and clear and one is never in doubt as to its interpretation.

Toward the end of her life when her sight was failing, she occasionally had secretarial help, and in 1891 she wrote to thank her friend William Rathbone for the loan of his Miss Stevens "as typewriter." Two years ago, I was privileged to meet Mrs. Alice Crawley, who had acted as Florence Nightingale's private secretary and companion from 1900 to 1904. Then 88 years old, Mrs. Crawley showed me a heart-shaped ring of emeralds and diamonds which Miss Nightingale gave to her, together with a check for 100 pounds on the eve of her wedding in 1904. Miss Cochrane, as she then was, was reluctant to leave her mistress, but the wise old lady divined the true state of affairs and told her that her sweetheart (who had lost an arm in the Boer War) needed her more than she did. Mrs. Crawley had vivid memories of the kindly octogenarian whose mind was still strong and nimble. She spent the greater part of the day in bed, but would get up to feed the birds on her balcony. One of Mrs. Crawley's main duties was to read the papers to Miss Nightingale, who missed nothing and made caustic comments on the politics and events of the day. It was easy to see that Miss Nightingale had made an indelible impression upon her, as she did indeed upon all who came in contact with her.

A great deal of that indefinable aura of greatness attaches to Miss Nightingale's letters. In them one sees her extraordinary versatility and intellectual power, her amazing grasp of things great and small, her ability to laugh—even at herself—the ease and the mastery in almost every line, whether she was writing to an elder statesman or a young probationer. Her humor was often sly. Writing to Dr. and Mrs. Howe in 1845, she reports that "the Queen is going to add a babby and Miss Martineau a book to the already numerous swarm." In 1867, she told her dentist that "I have broken four of my teeth lately, probably with gnashing them at ministers."

Her love of animals, especially cats, is constantly brought out. Writing to her friend Madame Mohl about an unexpected litter of kittens she says, "My cats will not have the husbands I choose, but take up with low Toms, of recent extraction, out of the mews." She frequently referred to her cats when ramming home matters of importance. In writing to the viceroy of India about sanitation (or rather the lack of it) in the Punjab, she says, "Medical officers are able to point out the evils, but they have no more clue to the remedies than my cats have."

Her sense of fun remained with her up to the end. In writing to Mrs. J. R. Green in 1894, she tells the story of the owl Athena which she had rescued from boys in the Parthenon in 1850 and brought back to England. "This favourite pet" she said, "dropped off his perch dead when he heard I was going to the Crimea."

Another striking trait is her consideration for her servants and dependents. Although she did not allow her name to be associated with any charity, her letters show that she gave anonymously to a great many causes, and her private benefactions to old soldiers and nurses were endless. Year after year letters of remembrance went out on birthdays and other anniversaries and they were invariably accompanied by gifts. For many years she paid the local doctors to attend the sick and aged villagers at Lea Hurst, her old family home in Derbyshire. She sent food, wine and whiskey, and characteristically, she catechized the doctors about their treatment and was not above suggesting some line of her own on occasions. To a domestic whose aunt was ill she writes, "Does she wear flannel next to the skin?" In 1873, she asks Dr. Sutherland about some pills which her maid Jenny is taking. "Would you believe it," she says, "that the maids of the supposed greatest authority on nursing take quack medicine?" Incidentally, although she made a slave of Dr. Sutherland, she was much attached to him. One of her innumerable letters to him had a postscript: "Your cold is very bad on your chest. Old Nurse." She could, on the other hand, be very bitter. Sir Douglas Galton was one of her most able and devoted "aides," but he was also an overworked undersecretary of state. Once, when he could not come to South Street at a time convenient to her, she wrote: "I must take the leavings, as beggars can't be choosers," and signed herself, "Your dog, F.N."

With reference to a list of questions that had been sent to her by the Matrons Council in 1895, she wrote, "It is rife with Preliminary Courses, Examinations, Theoretical Education, Certificates, State Registration, and so forth. I was glad to receive the sensible paper of the Bellevue Superintendent in the *Hospital* which does not go into all this farrago." She constantly tilts against the "certificate insanity" and against "the old superstition of infection," and she comments, "How strange it is that no woman between twenty and thirty now has any constitution."

And now, what of Florence Nightingale's message for today? First, in regard to the fundamentals of nursing, I think it is true to say that Florence Nightingale's prevision was such that no first principle laid down by her has needed alteration, or is likely to. The second lesson which we have to draw is that the extraordinary degree of success achieved by Miss Nightingale imposed certain limitations on the speed of further progress. This paradox could be paralleled in many other fields of social endeavor.

What was good enough for the great Florence Nightingale was to remain for many years good enough for all nurses, a life of unremitting toil, with devotion to one end, the care of the sick. Not so many years ago older members of the profession, in discussing charges that nursing hours were too long and conditions too arduous, were likely to give the reply: "In my day we did 84 hour a week," implying that what happened in their day was a standard to which any nurse who was really a nurse might be proud to work. I think a great disservice is done by those who thus misinterpret Miss Nightingale's teaching. Do they imagine that if Miss Nightingale were alive today she would not have changed her ideas?—not the fundamental principles, but her ideas regarding discipline and hours and conditions of work.

In 1893, a congress on hospitals, dispensaries, and nursing was held in connection with the famous World's Fair in Chicago. To the nursing section of this congress, Miss Nightingale sent a paper which is one of the most remarkable of all her writings. Her views on the nature of disease and on the role of the nurse in its control are staggering in their modernity:

> What is sickness? she asked. Sickness or disease is nature's way of getting rid of the effects of conditions which have interfered with health. It is nature's attempt to cure. We have to help her. Diseases are, practically speaking, adjectives, not noun substantives. What is health? Health is not only to be well, but to be able to use well every power we have. What is nursing? Both kinds of nursing are to put us in the best possible conditions for nature to restore or to preserve health, to prevent or to cure disease or injury. Upon nursing proper, under scientific heads, physicians or surgeons must depend partly, perhaps mainly, whether nature succeeds or fails in her attempts to cure by sickness. Nursing proper is therefore to help the patient suffering from disease to live, just as health nursing is to keep or put the constitution of the healthy child or human being in such a state as to have no disease.

Miss Nightingale devoted a great part of her address to the dangers that might arise after a generation of nursing. The greatest dangers she considered to be (1) fashion and its consequence of loss of earnestness, (2) mere money getting, and (3) making nursing a profession and not a calling. The last of the three is of course connected with her strong antipathy toward registration and certification of nurses, and here one can only say that her ideas would inevitably have changed with the development of the profession which she did in fact create. She referred to a further danger—perhaps the greatest of all—and here I think we come to the very essence of her message for today. The danger to which she referred was that of "stereotyping," not progressing:

> No system can endure that does not march. Are we walking to the future or to the past? Are we progressing or are we stereotyping? We remember that we have scarcely crossed the threshold of uncivilised civilisation in nursing: there is still so much to do. Don't let us stereotype mediocrity. We are still on the threshold of nursing.

In the future, which I shall not see, for I am old, may a better way be opened! May the methods by which every infant, every human being, will have the best chance of health, the methods by which every sick person will have the best chance of recovery, be learned and practised! Hospitals are only an intermediate stage of civilisation, never intended, at all events, to take in the whole sick population.

Many of the ideas to which Miss Nightingale gave such forcible expression in 1893 had been put forward 34 years earlier in her *Notes on Nursing*. She had always seen to the heart of things—that the real nurse must be a dedicated being—that the sick person must be treated and not the disease, that prevention is infinitely better than cure, that universal hospitalization will not give positive health, and that nursing must hold to its ideals but must change some of its methods—and now after a hundred years the ministers of health, the epidemiologists, and the psychosomatic experts are just beginning to catch up with her.

These two professors of Sociology received a grant from the United States Public Health Service's (USPHS) Division of Nursing to study the emerging professional identity among baccalaureate student nurses. Out of this project grew their interest in the socio-historical context of nursing. In this particular selection they apply the principles and conclusions common to the behavioral sciences in asking two questions: "Why did Florence Nightingale and not some other come to be regarded as the mother of nursing as a profession?" and "What was her unique contribution?" They answer that she left nursing a multi-faceted legacy of status and prestige that derived from her high social position and her own dramatic, even eccentric way of doing things. The perspective of the social scientist was thus added to the historiography surrounding Florence Nightingale.

ELVI WAIK WHITTAKER and VIRGINIA L. OLESEN

"Why Florence Nightingale?"

Nursing grants Florence Nightingale the status of originator, of culture heroine. It credits her with advocating a new ideology and with shaping the profile of the profession as it is today. That she and her work deserve the veneration and homage she is universally granted is not open to dispute. A closer examination of the socio-historical trends in nineteenth century England, however, lead one to reflect on the origins and development of the legend associated with her and to explore in greater detail the reasons why this particular woman emerged as the mother of the profession and not some one else?

This question presents itself with some force when certain facts are considered. She was far from being the first trained nurse, or even the creator of the first school of nursing. A system of training had been established some 200 years before her birth by St. Vincent de Paul in Paris, followed by others such as the one at Kaiserswerth in Germany and that of the Sisters of Charity in Ireland.

Neither was she the first to agitate for reforms in nursing or in hospitals. Pleas for this came repeatedly from eminent physicians, zealous clergy, and public-minded citizens alike. Nor was Florence Nightingale the first of her sex to direct her energies in this direction. There were women who had spent more years of their lives on behalf of nursing than had she, and many who worked toward the same ends as she at the very same time. Among them could be mentioned Amalie Sieveking, Felicia Skene, and the worthy Elizabeth Fry.

Nor was she the first lady of social stature to devote herself to social reform or to undertakings involving the lives of women. Here again the list is lengthy and includes illustrious women like Lady Mary Wortley Montague, Lady Hester Stanhope and Mary Wollstonecraft. Thus one still asks, why Florence Nightingale?

The answer must lie in the kind of woman Florence Nightingale was and the manner in which she set about her chosen tasks. In short, she was a woman of high status, and one who went about things in a dramatic way. Her adventure in the Crimea was an event which shattered forever the contemporary notions of what could and should be done by women. That she was a lady of the upper classes added impetus to the fervor with which the story was spread and applauded. It is difficult to appreciate the emotional and intellectual impact of her Crimean activities on Victorian England, where women were essentially second-class citizens, valued for their decorative and entertaining qualities, and for innocence of social and political issues.

With the aid of the London *Times*, the adventures of Florence Nightingale was spread to the literate population of England, and the story had an overwhelming appeal. The social milieu at the time was strongly colored by romanticism. Many a Victorian heart beat faster over tales of unrequited love, sacrifice, and tentavious virtue in the face of over-bearing odds, and the story of Florence Nightingale, the embodiment of all things brave and beautiful, found a natural place. A volume on world-noted women in 1857 included a chapter on Florence Nightingale, putting her in the prestigious company of Joan of Arc, St. Cecilia and Pocahontas, and more interestingly from a contemporary viewpoint, in the questionable company of Sappho, Cleopatra, and Catherine II.

So reverently and deferentially is she viewed that it is not entirely unusual to find members of the public uncertain whether she was real or a figure of myth or literature. In these misconceptions they are abetted by those who are themselves victims of incurable romanticism, who bestow on her qualities of saintliness, unremitting humility, absolute self-abnegation, and untainted innocence, which surely could only belong to persons above, and hence free from, the hurly-burly of human existence. Florence Nightingale's connection with nursing could only confer on the profession, and those who practiced it, some of the glory conferred on its powerful protagonist.

Not only romanticism, but also a renewed humanitarianism was woven into the social pattern of the nineteenth century. Obviously Florence Nightingale's deeds in the Crimea were the very essence of what was humane. The relatively comfortable sectors of English society were already imbued with the humanitarian spirit; and, as history will testify, while England at times presented the heights of industrial poverty and misery, it also advanced some of the most commendable reforms. The desperate and pitiable conditions of the wounded on the battlefields was by no means overlooked in this new fervor. Indeed, it was not entirely under her own impetus that Florence Nightingale took on herself the task of supervising nursing at Scutari; it resulted in part from the encouragement of Sidney Herbert, as head of the War Office, and the clergyman Henry Edward Manning (later Cardinal Manning), both of whom were sensitive to the urgent needs there.

Florence Nightingale, by being the stuff of which legends are made, invested nursing with themes which it hitherto lacked. Previously nursing had hardly been peopled by individuals who could appeal to the romantic and the humanitarian; this new heroine-nurse was able to lever the profession to the heights of social regard. These themes have persisted in the imagery of the profession, and, indeed, nursing itself has clung to them. Remnants of its nineteenth century past can be seen in tendencies even now to refer to the profession as a "calling," as one demanding sacrifice and self-denial. It can be seen in those segments of the profession that retain sentimentalized rituals like capping, notions of dedicating one's life and being "ministering angels."

Before Florence Nightingale, nursing was mainly in the hands of women who were certainly not noted for their high moral standards and many virtues. They could not even be noted for their sobriety. It is common to write of the degraded standards of nursing care at this time, mainly because this lends emphasis to the miraculous changes wrought through Florence Nightingale's efforts. Relatively little attention is given to the social situations that brought about the poor care.

Foremost among these is that work for women was tolerated only for those who needed the wages to feed themselves and their families. These women were poor, often abjectly poor. In addition, education for women was frowned on and consisted mainly in tutoring for the upper middle and upper classes. The tutoring was geared to helping genteel women acquire the "accomplishments" so highly esteemed at that time, and so necessary for establishing a respectable place in the courtship and marriage market, the only market for which women were destined. Hence it is not surprising that those nurses who were not attached to religious orders came from the poor laboring class. The position of governess was not open to them because of their lack of education and social status. They could, perhaps, aspire to an apprenticeship in millinery or dressmaking, or to domestic service. Yet, as these positions also were open only to women who could display some gentility, they were left with the choice of merciless hours in a factory or mine, where they were sometimes employed to do the work of a mule, or they could seek a position in a hospital.

It would have been difficult for Victorian England to associate humanism or romanticism with work done by women like these. In the interests of accuracy, however, while the images of Dickens' Sairey Gamp, of intoxication and theft, promiscuity and abuse, must describe some segments of the nursing population at that time, it could not be true for all. The following desription by a physician in a letter in the *London Times* of April 15, 1857, may be more apt:

Hospital nurses have for the last year or two been the victims of much unmerited abuse. They have their faults, but most of these may be laid to the want of proper treatment. Lectured by committees, preached at by chaplains, scowled on by treasurers and stewards, scolded by matrons, sworn at by surgeons, bullied by dressers, grumbled at and abused by patients; insulted if old and ill-favoured; talked flippantly to, if middle-aged and good-humoured; tempted and seduced, if young and well-looking,—they are just what any woman might be, exposed to the same influences,—meek, pious, saucy, careless, drunken, or unchaste, according to circumstances or temperament; but most attentive, and rarely unkind . . .

Indeed with some elasticity of imagination it is not entirely difficult to note some similarities on the nursing scene even today.

SOCIAL STATUS

Perhaps Florence Nightingale's greatest gift to nursing was her being, most decidedly, a woman from the upper classes; perhaps one could even say that she was a member of an untitled and landed aristocracy. The occupation of the males of this social group was to lead the life of a country gentleman, to spend one's time in pursuit of scholarship and foreign travel, as did William Nightingale, or to dabble in politics if so inclined. The Nightingale family enjoyed the same social status as many of the powerful and influential in politics and were acquainted with members of the Cabinet, the House of Lords and even the prime minister. Florence earned the sympathetic ear of Victoria herself. She had a status and political connections which exceeded most of the administrators and physicians with whom she had to deal.

Added to this social stature was an exceptional personality, extraordinary intelligence and energy, and an education equaled by very few women. Under her father's tutelage, Florence acquired no mean understanding of mathematics, science, and four modern languages, as well as Greek and Latin. Her scholarly publications ranged from a commendable and historic work on biostatistics to matters of religion and translations of Plato.

Although it is easy to see where the qualities of saintliness and supreme sacrifice became associated with her name, ironically it was rebellion, rather than anything else, that took Florence Nightingale to the Crimea. She rebelled against the stupidity and boredom of the feminine life style of Victorian England. While the sentimentally enslaved nineteenth century described her as self-abnegating, humble, and saintly, modern history pictures her as peppery, obstinate, rageful, and demanding.

The latter portrait, coupled with the authority conferred by her upper class status, makes much more sense. It explains how she was able to pester and demand, to cajole and manipulate to accomplish that on which she had set heart and mind—and usually this was on a grand scale involving the higher reaches of Parliamentary affairs. Nursing, one of the many reforms on which she showered her attention, benefited greatly. She dealt effectively with shortsighted physicians at Scutari and doubting members of the government at home. Saintliness could hardly suffice to accomplish this. Rather, fire and determination, the cold and ruthless use of status and power were her weapons.

EMANCIPATION

Florence Nightingale, her status and deeds, played a leading role in the general movement to emancipate women, although she always shirked connections with the movement and was, in essence, opposed to it. And small wonder. From her vantage point she already had great power, without emancipation. Through her example women became somewhat more liberated, somewhat freer to seek occupation outside the home. Not only did nursing acquire higher status because she was associated with it, but also nurses, as such, became more respectable. The almost caste-like social system of England had prohibited women of the upper strata from demeaning themselves with work, for the social and physical condition of these women was seen as the outward reflection of a man's success and financial position. They served somewhat the same function in this respect as that occupied today by costly or rare pets. A wife's idleness was directly related to a man's importance, and even the very garb of ladies of fashion reflected the life they were expected to lead:

The small hand, and therefore the tight glove, indicated that the owner was above having to do manual work; the huge crinoline signified that the wearer occupied a large space in the social world, the trailing skirt that she did not belong to the "walking classes," and the stiff corset that she was a woman of unbending rectitude . . . May we not also read in the small waist a mute appeal for the support of the masculine arm?

The growing and relatively wealthy middle class followed the example of ladies of "accomplishment" and "cultivation," and, as is ever the pattern in matters of status, were meticulous in doing what the upper classes deemed appropriate, while at the same time effectively keeping women of the lower social orders "in their place." It is interesting to note, *à propos* of this, that the words, "snobbish" and "respectable" acquired their present meanings during the nineteenth century.

Inevitably many a lady, many a daughter of the "comfortable," railed against such enforced idleness, the weakness and innocence so admired by Victorian manhood. And undoubtedly many were made exceedingly unhappy by the prisons, in the guise of Victorian marriages, based as they were on denials of individuality, the avoidance of intelligent conversations, and the espousal of child-like innocence.

Had Florence married Richard Monckton Milnes (later Lord Houghton), as she at one point contemplated, her life would have been quite different, revolving less around voluminous writings and heroic deeds, and more around the counting of household silver and linen, the

appropriate appearances at social gatherings, and the occasional, usually patronizing, visits to the poor and the sick. An interesting contem-
plation for the nursing historian is: what themes would have become
part of the nursing story, and how would nursing have evolved without
Florence Nightingale?

At the same time, nursing reforms instigated by Florence offered
a solution to women of the lower classes, who undeniably needed to
earn their own living—and that of their numerous dependents—and to
do it in a manner that could afford them some semblance of decency.
They needed to be freed from occupations which afforded them only
cellar rooms perpetually crowded and moist from inefficient drainage
in London streets. They needed to see meat on their tables if only once
a week. They needed to save their children from the far too early on-
slaught of menial and crippling work and the prospects of nothing but
a poverty like that of their parent. These women undoubtedly cast
covetous eyes at the respectability and comforts of those in the social
class above them. Florence Nightingale and the new body of nurses,
trained and respectable, suggested an answer.

While slowly advancing feminine emancipation provided the appropriate social climate, Florence Nightingale set the dramatic example.
Being of a status that even most "ladies" would find desirable, she
suggested an avenue whereby women of status could capitalize on all
the romantic and humanitarian values of the times and become heroines
by involving themselves with the nursing of the sick. The idle could
escape from boredom, the intelligent from feigned naiveté. Florence
provided for them in her outline of a training system for nursing
under a category of "lady nurses," which was to include women of
serious intent and a willingness to devote their energies to the profession.

On the other hand she opened the door as well to the wage-earning
group of women, offering them training and the possibility of an
elevated status, such as would come to them through working with
women of higher station, in a profession that was rapidly earning
public respect. Hence social mobility and "respectability" became
realities for them.

Nursing can trace some of its present status and prestige to this
woman, who chose to forego the comfortable and wearisome existence
Victorian life offered her, to etch out for herself a role far different
from that prescribed by society. Undoubtedly she was an eccentric,
but as such she was able to leave nursing a many-faceted legacy. By
association with a woman of such status and such dramatic and

legendary accomplishment, professional nursing acquired romantic and humanitarian overtones and a respectable social stature.

This "Occasional Paper" by a British nurse administrator was selected by the British Medical Association as a Prize-winning Essay in 1968. In it, Florence Nightingale is viewed as the prime mover and at times even the "sole architect" of many late nineteenth century reforms. Reflecting a keen awareness of earlier work, Baly opens: "Florence Nightingale was a legend in her own day, but no miasma of sentimentality nor subsequent reaction of anti-myth can destroy the solid facts of her achievements: they were Herculean." Nevertheless, the author challenges her profession as it enters the 1970's to cease living "in the shadow of a legend." In her words, "Miss Nightingale adapted her system to the needs and the changing attitudes of the 1860's; she gave us a springboard not a mattress; principles, not ossified rules. If we cannot adapt the fault is ours, not hers."

MONICA E. BALY

"Florence Nightingale's Influence on Nursing Today"

The Greatest Victorian

Mrs. Cecil Woodham Smith described Miss Nightingale as 'The Greatest Victorian of them all'; as there are so many eminent Victorians it is a large claim, but it is difficult to fault. Florence Nightingale was a legend in her own day, but no miasma of sentimentality nor subsequent reaction of anti-myth can destroy the solid facts of her achievements; they were Herculean.

For the best part of 50 years she laboured unremittingly 'for the sake of the work', using every weapon she had to achieve her purpose, and her weapons were many: a first-class intellect, a passion for statistics, influence in high places, royal patronage, charm, a talent for the incisive aphorism, and above all the imagination to see what needed to be done. In the débâcle of the Crimean War her achievements shine like a beacon, but it was not in nursing alone that she effected reform; the hygiene of barracks, the diet of the army, recreational facilities for soldiers, military clothing, the files of the India Office, all came under her scrutiny and were the subject of her pungent reports.

She said she had 'lived through Hell' and her life's work was to see that such preventable suffering did not happen again; she knew that every day reform was delayed people were dying unnecessarily.

Although Miss Nightingale was the prime mover, and in some cases the sole architect of many reforms in the second part of the 19th century, they can all be seen against this background: the desire to prevent suffering. In reforming nursing it is for this reason her efforts were bent not only to the hospital but to prevention of ill-health in the community.

After her return from the Crimea Miss Nightingale set her hand to two major reforms, The Health, Efficiency and Hospital Administration in the British Army, and a reform of hospital nursing. In spite of opposition, frustration and dark despair, in both she triumphed, and both had far-reaching effects. It is debatable who owes most to Miss Nightingale: the British Army or nursing.

Reform of Nursing

Although Miss Nightingale's reforms eventually covered hospitals, Poor Law Institutions, midwifery and nursing in the community, her most spectacular reform was in hospital nursing. In this she laid the foundations of modern nursing and gave this country and many others a system that has stood the test of a century.

The background to her reforms was her own practical experience in the Crimea where her efforts to provide a nursing service with the available material had been so nearly wrecked by the disputes of the religious orders and the ignorance and indiscipline of some of the hospital nurses. She had learnt in the hard school the need for a corps of intelligent and trained women who had, as their first duty, the care of the sick and not the proselytizing for a particular creed.

The second half of the century was ripe for reform; evangelical and liberal thought was changing the public attitude to poverty and disease, medical knowledge was advancing and the voluntary hospitals had been expanding for over 100 years. At the same time intelligent women were beginning to rebel against the Victorian strait-jacket of enforced feminine uselessness.

Miss Nightingale's objective was to secure intelligent women who would act as skilled auxiliaries to the doctors and who would be capable of handling, supervising and reporting accurately on the patients under their care. To attain this objective she knew she must select carefully and train rigorously. The money donated by a grateful public in recognition of her services in the Crimea gave her the opportunity to put into practice her carefully thought out experiment.

It was not, however, an experiment that had universal approbation; there was opposition on all sides, particularly from the doctors. Mr. South, the senior consultant surgeon at St. Thomas's, where the experiment was to take place, wrote that they were 'not at all disposed to allow that the nursing establishments of our hospitals are inefficient or that they are likely to be improved by any special institution for nursing'. He argued that nurses were subordinates 'in the position of housemaids'.

Because of this atmosphere of hostility it was essential that the first probationers should be above suspicion; the whole enterprise depended on them. They must be 'the incarnate denial that a hospital nurse needed to be drunken and promiscuous'. The scheme must therefore allay hostility and gain public acceptance. The discipline of the first Nightingale school was not discipline for discipline's sake; it was there to secure approval for the system. The triad of the plan was training of the character, the acquisition of skill and knowledge, and nursing administration in the hands of nurses—a triad which even the most radical reformers would not wish to deny 100 years later.

To achieve these objectives, carefully selected pupils of good education and moral standing did a year's training in the Nightingale School, living in a 'home' supervised by a home sister. The 'nurses' home' was an innovation of Miss Nightingale's divising; it reflected the cultural pattern of her own home and was designed to inculcate these values into the probationers. It also ensured strict supervision so that no breath of scandal could assail the Nightingale ladies.

Although Miss Nightingale envisaged her training as suitable for any intelligent girl of the right aptitude and character, the scheme attracted daughters of the upper class. After seven years there developed two methods of entry: one for ordinary probationers who did a two-year training and who received free maintenance, uniform and a £10 allowance, and the other, a one-year training, for 'lady probationers', who paid for their training.

It was not Miss Nightingale's intention to restrict entry to one class, but the ladies helped to supplement the finances of the Nightingale Fund, and after a while Miss Nightingale appreciated the leadership qualities they could bring to what was a missionary campaign. Eventually this system gave way to a standard two-year training, but it left its mark on the profession. Other hospitals with strained resources copied it whole or in part; even in the 1930s it was not uncommon for entrants to pay for their uniform and for the preliminary training school. The ability of parents to bear part of the cost had a social cachet which in turn led to a dichotomy, one of the many historical factors that had led to disunity in nursing.

The economic rewards and training patterns were set, and were to last in the main principles for a century.

Nursing Administration

Miss Nightingale was quite clear about her aims. She wrote:

> 'The whole reform of nursing both at home and abroad has consisted of this: to take the power over nursing out of the hands of the men and to put it into the hands of one female trained head and make her responsible for everything (regarding internal management and discipline) being carried out'.

Unless she achieved this objective the experiment failed. No one was more meticulous than Miss Nightingale in insistence on absolute obedience to the orders of the doctor as far as treatment was concerned. But nursing was more than just blind obedience and technical skill, it was intelligent comfort and care, trained observation and doing for the patient those things he could not do for himself.

Much ink has been spilled on 'the proper task of the nurse', but for guidance we could do worse than look at *Notes on Nursing* and other writings of Miss Nightingale; these astringent comments still have relevance even in a world of heart and lung transplants. We might start with: 'It is the first duty of the hospital that it shall do the patient no harm'.

To achieve the practice of nursing as an art it was absolutely necessary that nurses and would-be nurses were administered by someone who understood that art. Nurses were there to nurse. In any event the supervision of nurses by doctors, chaplains and lay administrators in the previous half century had hardly shown commendable results.

In order to achieve this change the Nightingale School became a power house for training matrons. Promising pupils were sent forth as missionaries; they had been trained to train. Such was the fame of the Nightingale School that the services of its trainees were eagerly sought, although once in their new posts they were not always so eagerly welcomed. Many were the battles that ensued between the old and the new. The new Nightingales set about their reforming with a zeal worthy of Miss Nightingale herself; in spite of setbacks, invariably at the end of the day they triumphed. The new matrons had carved themselves an empire.

Reforms in Poor Law Institutions

Although nursing reform in the voluntary hospitals was the most spectacular, the reforms in the Poor Law Institutions were perhaps more far-reaching. The need was more desperate and they affected more people. In 1869 there were about 50,000 sick paupers living in institutions that were designed, not to care for the sick, but to implement the less eligibility test. Care, if any, was in the hands of pauper nurses.

Louisa Twining had already exposed the evils in the London work-houses, and William Rathbone, a Liverpool philanthropist, enlisted Miss Nightingale's help in starting a nursing service in the institution at Brownlow Hill. The battle for reform in the conditions of sick paupers was even more formidable than the battle in the voluntary hospitals. At least the hospitals had a tradition of philanthropy; the work-houses were there to deter. The upper class reformers spoke the same language as the governors of hospitals; the boards of guardians did not.

Reform was long, bitter and often disappointing. Miss Nightingale never achieved complete success, but the experiment of using trained nurses at Brownlow Hill and elsewhere proved the point; eventually, in the years between the Metropolitan Poor Law Act in 1867 and the Royal Commission on Poor Law 1909, the system of using separate infirmaries staffed with trained nurses, albeit often sparsely, became almost universal.

Nevertheless, although the system of training became universal the type of entrant did not; the tradition of the Poor Law hung like a veil for many years, providing a curtain between 'voluntary hospital nurses' and 'municipal nurses'.

District Nursing

In 1861 William Rathbone drew Miss Nightingale's attention to the need for nursing care for the poor who were sick in their own homes. He had already tried an experiment of his own but could not pursue it because of lack of suitable nurses. After much consideration Miss Nightingale concluded that the only hope was to train nurses specially for the purpose. At William Rathbone's expense Liverpool Royal Infirmary started a training school for nurses; a percentage of the trainees was reserved for the hospital and the remainder went to work on the district.

It was the forerunner of other similar schemes, and, in spite of the crushing burden of the other work, Miss Nightingale always kept the threads of district training in her own hands; there was no equivocation about their duties, they were not almsgivers, they were not doctors, they were there to give trained nursing care.

In 1887 Queen Victoria decided to devote part of the Women's Jubilee Gift to the cause of nursing the poor in their own homes, and Miss Nightingale persuaded the trustees that the best way of doing this was to train nurses. Thus the Jubilee Institute for Nurses was founded, and trained nursing care in the community ran *pari passu* to that in the hospitals.

Health Visiting

Notes on Nursing precede the germ theory of infection, yet with an almost incredible perspicacity they foreshadow it. 'Lack of proper health teaching' is the theme. Florence Nightingale said once: 'I look to the day when there will be no nurses of the sick, only nurses to the well'.

Prevention is the keynote to all her writings and teachings. In 1892 when she was living at Claydon with the Verneys she had a chance to put into operation a scheme she had long cherished: the idea that there should be a corps of health missionaries to support the work of the district nurses. With the help of Sir Harry Verney and the North Bucks Technical Education Committee, a course was started for suitable educated women to be trained as teachers of health. These forerunners of our health visitors so established themselves that by 1909 their training was governed by statute. They were to form the basis for an important and unique part of British nursing.

Miss Nightingale's Influence on Nursing in the 20th Century

One test of the enduring influence of the reforms effected by Miss Nightingale is to ask to what extent they have affected the development of nursing in this country and abroad. There can be no gainsaying that the effect has been profound, and of all the influences on nursing it has been the most healthy.

Influence on Nurse Training

The main tenets of the Nightingale system have been an article of faith for the nursing profession. However, much that has passed for the 'Nightingale system' has traduced the intentions of Miss Nightingale herself. First, she was a superb statistician; she knew that all sick persons could not be nursed by her highly trained and carefully selected nurses. They were trained to train and to supervise the existing nurses, and by supervision make them better nurses.

But the system was caught in the web of its own success. The prestige conferred on a hospital in having a training school for nurses, and the apparently unending stream of devoted young women offering themselves, led more hospitals to start training schools. Soon the criterion became, not the production of trained nurses to be sent forth to train others, but a supply of biddable probationers who would form the major part of the nursing service, or when trained would remain on the staff.

Secondly, the lady probationers, whom Miss Nightingale had reluctantly accepted, became the first matrons. Lacking the practical sense of their founder they sought to restrict nursing to upper class entrants, hoping to demand a high qualifying examination, not to mention a swingeing registration fee. Illogically they would not entertain the idea of more than one grade of nurse.

The corollary was obvious: if the increasing demand for nurses was to be met, and there was only to be one grade and one qualifying examination, then the selection and standard must be lowered. Ostrich-like for over 40 years the nursing profession refused to face its options. The influence, however, was not Miss Nightingale's but Mrs. Bedford Fenwick's. This influence on the profession, on doctors and administrators, can be seen in the almost fanatical resistance in some quarters to the introduction of a shorter training for the assistant nurse and to the Nurses' Act of 1943.

It is not the influence of the original Nightingale training on nursing that has caused the havoc, but the departure from it. The Nightingale School in 1860 was financed independently by the Nightingale Fund. Although the probationers undoubtedly contributed to the service of the hospital, their training needs came first. This has been the main recommendation of every report on nurse training from Horder to Platt, including the Government's own report on The Recruitment and Training of Nurses, 1948. 'Reports are not self-executive' wrote Miss Nightingale. They are not.

Are the original principles of the Nightingale scheme still valid? Obviously the simple but rigorous training of 1860 is not suitable for the complexities of medical knowledge in the second half of the 20th century, but even the suggestion for nurse training in A Comprehensive Medical Education that a basic degree in human biology would be a suitable foundation for some nurse training would not deny these principles. In a time of rapid expansion and evaluation of degree courses for nurses, the acquisition of knowledge and skill are the right principles for nurse training.

The Nurses' Home

The Nightingale Home had a specific purpose: to give a cultural background and to supervise personal behaviour. Once the experiment was a success, provided selection was high, rigorous discipline was no longer necessary. In subsequent years the provision of a nurses' home, except in the more wealthy hospitals, was not to provide a cultural background, but to keep a large trainee labour force close at hand for the long and often unsocial hours they were required to work. There seems little evidence that later home sisters spent time discussing poetry with their charges.

Much has been made of the early discipline and its effect, but the first probationers were invited to criticize their lectures, an exercise in participative management that has not had much place in the intervening years. Although nurses' homes are becoming white elephants, the latest body to pronounce on nurses, the Prices and Incomes Board, recommends that student nurses should live in during their first year, which was all Miss Nightingale originally asked.

Nursing Administration

The Nightingale reforms brought a revolution to hospital administration. The matron became the supreme head of the nursing services and the training school. It gave us our so-called and often maligned tripartite administration. There is, however, no evidence to suggest that mere dual administration would have been easier. Indeed, the unseemly acrimony of the 19th century dual system makes our present little local difficulties pale into insignificance. The idea that the matron should be head of the training school is embedded in the nursing profession as Holy Writ; the shocked horror at the suggestion in the Wood Report that nurse training should be under the control of a training authority and not a hospital is evidence of this.

The Report on Senior Nursing Staff Structure (Salmon) in 1967 was careful to leave this principle inviolate; the chief nursing officer (Grade 10) is head of all nursing services and training within the ambit of her group. Is this too much for one person? Will the future of nurse education perforce be more closely linked with outside educational bodies? Is this one Nightingale principle that we must eventually throw overboard? One feels Miss Nightingale would not mind provided the profession kept control of its own education.

The Report on Senior Nursing Staff Structure has in fact shattered the idea that the matron must be the supreme head. With a layer of 'top management' having structural authority over 'matrons' of units, the old concept is dead. Nevertheless, the principle remains; what Miss Nightingale fought for was that one trained nurse should be in charge of all nursing matters. One doubts if she would have minded whether it was a hospital or a group, a matron or a chief nursing officer. If the Committee had recommended that someone *other* than a nurse should be in charge of the nursing services, then well might we have wrung our hands and said, 'The spirit of Nightingale is dead'.

Pay and Conditions of Service

Traditionally nurses were always rewarded partly in kind. The Nightingale system undoubtedly set the seal on this. Once the comforts of a Victorian upper class home were supplied, all that was needed was pocket money, and preferably a private income, a not unexceptionable method of reward in 1860. The difficulty came in the years between the wars when many nurses' homes did not provide upper class comforts and when private incomes were no more.

The battle to remove nurses from this system is hardly won. Traditional public and management thinking is still the picture of a nurse as a young, single, dedicated woman, not a married man, a widow with children, a woman supporting parents or even just herself until death parts her from her small pension.

Miss Nightingale's Influence on the General Development of British Nursing

By amazing prescience Miss Nightingale gave to us not only reformed professional hospital nursing, but a nursing service to the community backed by a special corps of nurses trained to prevent ill-health—the forerunners of our health visitors. Countries which did not adopt the Nightingale system have poorly developed community nursing and preventive services. In order to provide a child welfare service for the displaced persons camps in Germany in 1948, it was necessary to start our own training on British lines; the concept of positive child health services was unknown.

Underdeveloped countries have wanted from us not so much hospital nurses but highly trained public health nurses; a poor country needs not expensive hospitals, but health. This has been a unique British contribution to world health, a contribution that owes its origin to Miss Nightingale's first lady health missionaries. Although much still needs to be done to integrate the work of hospitals and the health services to the community, at least the Nightingale reforms gave us a comprehensive nursing service.

The Influence of Tradition on Nursing

The achievements of reform in the second half of the 19th century cannot be minimized. They are legendary. However, living in the shadow of a legend is not an unmitigated blessing. Exhorted to the 'Nightingale spirit', praised as 'ministering angels', sicklied o'er with pale cast of sentimentality, nurses have tended to cling blindly to the tradition that raised them to such a pinnacle. To question the system was *lèse-majesté*, and this bred orthodoxy; conformity operates against reform. In spite of some enlightened questioning, the profession has tended to look back to its days of glory and has chosen not reform, but a crown of thorns.

Nursing, once saved by an outstanding woman, has had an almost Messianic belief that this would happen again. But no new Nightingale will arise; this is not the need of the 20th century. The profession has it in its own hands to match the hour. Miss Nightingale adapted her system to the needs and the changing attitudes of the 1860s; she gave us a springboard, not a mattress; principles, not ossified rules. If we cannot adapt the fault is ours, not hers.

The author is professor of nursing at the Yale School of Nursing and professor of public health and chief of the Division of Health Services Administration at Yale University. This article is a fuller version of the Sybil Palmer Bellow Lecture presented by the author at the Yale School of Nursing in April, 1977. Because it is primarily an examination of Miss Nightingale's beliefs and actions as they relate to the nurse's position within the present health care system, the article is ideal as a closing selection. As viewed by Thompson, the dilemma—"whether nursing is a profession in and of itself, or whether nursing is a means to develop a better health care delivery system—lies at the heart of the two faces Florence Nightingale has presented to posterity."

JOHN D. THOMPSON

"The Passionate Humanist: From Nightingale to the New Nurse"

In times of radical change, there is an irrepressible desire to return to one's beginnings, to the history or genesis of the concepts undergoing change. This urge was dramatically illustrated recently by the phenomenal public participation in the television series based on *Roots*.

Such a recourse to history has both an intellectual and therapeutic reward. This history of ideas and the changes in these ideas—in our particular case, the changes in the practice of nursing—is a fascinating subject. Although an examination of our professional genes must be a continuous one to include newer knowledge and developments, it is not my intention to approach these changes in nursing from a revisionist point of view. Rather, I aim to probe the myths of our beginnings a little more deeply and, above all, to examine the truth of the two stereotypes by which Miss Nightingale has been categorized and in terms of which our profession has often been viewed. That these stereotypes persist even today is illustrated, on the one hand, by the poster of a pristinely clean and beautiful nurse with a finger over her lips urging visitors to be quiet in the hospital and, on the other hand, by the emasculatingly cruel character of head nurse Ratchet in *One Flew Over the Cuckoo's Nest*.

It is possible that such an intellectual reconsideration may have its therapeutic side effects as well. From any treatment process we learn that insight, increased general understanding, and a sense of continuity are valuable therapeutic modalities, particularly in times of personal stress. To carry the personal/professional analogy a bit further, it is possible that a review of the beginnings of our profession may alleviate the fears of those undergoing professional distress as a result of changes, many of which are regarded by some members of the profession as heresies.

No one can doubt that changes are occurring in nursing. One may not be able to determine too precisely what the "new nurse" is, but one can certainly determine that whatever she is, it is different from what she was. One of the problems in defining this "new nurse" is that one can classify the "newness" in several categories; there is even a lack of internal consistency within and between these emerging roles. An additional complication is that some of these changes are not solely in the hands of the profession itself, but have been influenced in recent years by a much broader social movement—i.e., the changing role of women in society. It is necessary, therefore, to tease out at least some of these changes in order to relate them to their origins.

The "new nurse" is partly an outcome of the nurse practitioner or nurse clinician movement, which proposes to extend the nurse's responsibility to include broader clinical and counseling functions in her relationship to the patient and his family. This, of course, impinges on certain areas of practice formerly considered the exclusive property of physicians or social workers.

In addition, there is the "primary nurse" concept, which changes the relationship between the nurse and the patient. It does so not necessarily in terms of the expansion of the nurse's clinical role (although this is a part of it), but in that it transfers to the nurse the responsibility and authority for the individual patient's care as it is provided by others as well as herself. The establishment of a meaningful therapeutic relationship includes the ability to delegate some responsibilities while still maintaining control.

The third area of change lies in the spectrum of technical skills that the nurse is now expected to possess. These technical achievements may or may not be directly affected by her role as clinician or primary nurse practitioner, and there may be no change at all in her relationship to other health care professionals, but she is expected to be able to read and interpret EKGs, handle a variety of intravenous feedings and medications, and interpret rather complex laboratory data. How she uses these skills depends upon her specific role definition.

In short, the new nurse has heightened responsibilities in addition to her redefined role and critical interrelationships with the individual patient. There is a strong bond between these newer professional roles, on the one hand, and broader nurse involvement in the total health care delivery system, on the other. For unless nurses can effectively bring about change in the way health care is evaluated and delivered in this country, their new roles may never emerge from the inadequacies, illogical contraints, and irrational decision options which now characterize both the system itself and the nurse's role within it.

The nursing profession is in a strong position to make these changes, not only because it is the largest health care profession, but because new modes of entry into the decision-making arenas are now open to nurses as a result of recent Federal legislation. Many of these programs present new and almost unique opportunities for nursing to make its presence felt in the design of the future health care delivery system. However, such opportunities also present nurses with a dilemma: Should they consolidate, develop, and enrich their new professional roles *apart* from the delivery system? Or should they turn their attention to analyzing and proposing changes in the system and then fashioning their new roles *within* the redesigned system?

Let me restate the two positions to make them clearer. On the one hand, the group I will call *professionalists* hold that: 1) nursing has been dominated too long by physicians, hospital administrators, health planners, and the like; 2) there is ample evidence from recent studies that the nurse functioning in an expanded role can make positive contributions to high quality health care; 3) first priority, therefore, must be given to consolidating these new roles and strengthening the right of the profession to determine its own future; and 4) whatever changes do occur in the delivery system, the new nurse will have become, by then, a force that must be dealt with.

The second group, whom I will call the *synergists,* would agree with the first two propositions. But they would hold as their third that the constraints of the present system limit the effectiveness of nurses—even those in expanded roles—in meeting patients' needs. And, as their fourth proposition, the synergists would hold that nursing's first priority should be to alter that system, because nurses will be unable to make their optimal contribution until substantive changes have been made in the total health care system.

This dilemma—whether nursing is a profession in and of itself, or whether nursing is a means to develop a better health care delivery system—lies at the heart of the two faces Florence Nightingale has presented to posterity.

Florence Nightingale returned to London from the Crimea on August 5, 1856, one year and nine months after she landed at Scutari and climbed the hill to the Barrack Hospital. She sneaked back to England disguised as a Miss Smith in the company of her aunt and a Queen's messenger. The stealthy re-entry was necessary because of threatened receptions—rides through triumphal arches accompanied by the bands of the Coldstream Guards, the Grenadiers, and the Fusiliers. She needed rest, she said.

She was already famous. Three months before, in his last appearance in the House of Lords, Lord Ellsmere had described his countrymen's esteem:

> The vegetation of two springs has obscured the vestiges of Balaclava and Inkerman. The ranks are full, the hospitals empty. The angel of mercy still lingers to the last on the scene of her labours, but her mission is all but accomplished. Those long arches of Scutari in which dying men sat up to catch the sound of her footsteps or the flutter of her dress, and fell back content to have seen her shadow as it passed, are now completely deserted.

Lord Stanley assessed her influence differently. "Mark what, by breaking through custom and prejudices, Miss Nightingale has effected for her sex. She has opened for them a new profession, a new sphere of usefulness." Her most complete biographer, E.T. Cook, stated that "she had come back from the East more resolved than ever to be a pioneer in the reform of nursing."

But that must wait: first, she intended to use her reputation and experience to reform the British army's medical service. She would not allow the spring vegetation to obscure her memories of the men who had needlessly died in those battles. Cecil Woodham-Smith describes her state of mind upon her return most succinctly: "She was a haunted woman, but she was pursued not by ghosts, but by facts, the facts of preventable disease."

She started with the Queen, whom she met on September 15th, to request a Royal Commission to inquire into the conditions of the army at the Crimea. With her ally, Mr. Herbert, she wrote out the instructions for the commission and selected its membership. When delay followed delay on the part of both the prime minister and the war office, she wrote her own report entitled, "Notes Affecting the Health, Efficiency, and Hospital Administration of the British Army," in a period of only six months. It was never published, although much of it was included in the eventual Royal Commission report.

The commission was finally set up in April, 1857; its findings were to be reported in three months. Miss Nightingale was not appointed a member, and even Strachey, hardly her admirer, intimated that this was unfair. "Today (1918) she would, of course, have been one of the Commission herself; but at that time the idea of a woman appearing in such a capacity was unheard of, and no one even suggested the possibility of Miss Nightingale's doing so." At any rate, it is widely recognized that she, Mr. Herbert, and Dr. Southerland wrote the report. Miss Nightingale limited her formal contribution to the submission of written testimony in answer to written questions, and there is much evidence that she supplied other questions for the commission members to use in their cross-examination of witnesses.

While all this rather frenetic activity was going on, she also radically altered the architecture of hospitals, having been asked to comment on the construction of a new army hospital at Netley. There she laid down the foundations of the pavilion plan that would influence hospital architecture for nearly a century. But more important, it was at this time that she began to develop a most unfeminine weapon— the use of statistics.

It is in a letter written in 1857 to an unknown correspondent that the real basis for Miss Nightingale's future strategy can be found. The letter points out,

> We had during the first seven months of the Crimean campaign a mortality among the troops at the rate of 60 percent per annum from disease alone, the rate of mortality which exceeds that of the great plague in London and a higher ratio than the mortality in cholera to the attacks. We had during the last six months of the war a mortality among our sick not much more than among our healthy guards at home and a mortality among our troops in the last five months two-thirds only of what it is among our troops at home.

Here she was reporting the results of one of the most successful research efforts ever made in army hygiene. She was also pointing out that if it were possible to have a lower mortality in the Crimea than in Great Britain, then something must be wrong in Great Britain.

Shortly after Miss Nightingale's return from the Crimea, she met Dr. William Farr and was able to apply his mortality tables to those of the army. This relationship with Dr. Farr continued to be a close one for some time, and there is much evidence that he was also actively involved in the report of the Royal Commission.

Miss Nightingale did not rush into statistics blindly, although she had a strong intuitive sense of their meaning. Few books made a greater impression on her than those of Adolph Quetelet, the Belgian statistician. This is reported by Cook, who devotes an entire chapter to describing her as "The Passionate Statistician." No one was more aware than Miss Nightingale of the inaccuracies of the mortality and morbidity statistics kept by the British Army; in fact, a complete section of the report of the Royal Commission was directed to the formation of a statistical department within the army. However, the army was not her only target. She soon directed her attention to the hospitals in London.

The degree of her insight into the problems of applying the statistical model to civilian hospitals was remarkable. In 1857, early in the formulation of her analytic model, and after reviewing the mortality statistics of the London hospitals, she wrote to Farr:

> You would, however, derive great joy and satisfaction for the one fact they point out is that the mortality increases as the number of patients. There are some differences between the hospitals which, however, can be explained by some taking in worse cases than others. 7.9 deaths in every 100 cases treated is the general rate in general hospitals, 9.38 in workhouses, 11.48 in special hospitals. The rest of my agreeable information I defer till I have the pleasure of seeing you again.

There are two remarkable features of this letter. The first is her use of the terms "joy and satisfaction" and "agreeable information" in describing mortality rates. (Is it any wonder Cook used the adjective "passionate" in describing her approach to this aspect of her endeavors? Or that I have paraphrased him, with equal accuracy, in the title of this article?) The joy came not from the subject matter, but rather from the fact that she had unearthed new knowledge that the larger the hospital, the higher the mortality. The second is that she recognized this early that the factor of differences in case mix between hospitals must be accounted for, and she immediately addressed herself to this awesome problem.

In 1860, she presented to the International Statistical Conference a proposed hospital statistical system that contained the seed of the now widely accepted international classification of diseases. This system was almost a revolutionary idea at the time, and we have not even yet succeeded in accomplishing the objectives she so carefully laid out when she proposed it. Her concepts translate readily into the techniques used today in utilization review, both for admission and for lengths of stay, medical care evaluation studies, and studies of cost effectiveness and cost benefit.

Under the concept of utilization review, she points out:

> It is a rule without any exception that no patients ought ever to stay a day longer than is absolutely essential for medical or surgical treatment.

In Section IX, where she presents her statistical system, she deals with the institutional effect of utilization review:

> The relation of the duration of cases to the general utility of the hospital has never been shown although it is obvious that if, by any sanitary means or improved treatment, the duration of cases could be reduced to one-half, the utility of the hospital would be doubled as far as its funds are concerned.

and she continues,

> They (statistics) would enable us to ascertain . . . what diseases and ages press most heavily on the resources of particular hospitals. For example, it was found that a very large proportion of the limited finances of one hospital was swallowed up by one preventable disease—Rheumatism,—to the exclusion of many important cases or other diseases from the benefits of the hospital treatment.

With regard to medical care quality evaluation, she states,

> (The proposed forms) would enable the mortality in hospitals, and also the mortality from particular diseases, injuries, and operations, to be ascertained with accuracy; and these facts, together with the duration of cases, would enable the value of particular methods of treatment and of special operations to be brought to statistical proof.

As far as cost effectiveness is concerned, she says,

> These statistics would show subscribers how their money was being spent,

what amount of good was really being done with it, or whether the money was doing mischief rather than good.

The cost benefit approach is contained in a phrase:

They (statistical methods) would enable us to ascertain the mortality in different hospitals, as well as from different diseases and injuries at the same and at different ages, the relative frequency of different diseases and injuries among the classes which enter hospitals in different countries, and in different districts of the same country. They could enable us to ascertain how much of each year of life is wasted by illness.

It is interesting to review that section of *Eminent Victorians* which contains her biography, as well as a lesser known volume by Greenwood entitled *Some British Pioneers of Social Medicine*. What is evident is the change in tone of the authors when they are discussing Miss Nightingale's work in nursing and when they are discussing her work on hospitals, with the commission, or in the area of social reform. Greenwood calls her "no scientist" (he also points out that Strachey was neither a scientist nor an administrator), although he is speaking from a post-Pierson era when the real science of statistics was born. However, he admits that she used statistics effectively. In comparing her with her friend, Chadwick, the great sanitary reformer in England, Greenwood says,

Among these earlier pioneers of whom I have written at length, Chadwick had the nearest likeness to Florence Nightingale. Of course, there are great differences. In the Victorian sense of the words, Florence Nightingale was a lady, but Chadwick, hardly a gentleman. Both were bitter critics, but one used a neater weapon of offense than the other, a rapier not a bludgeon. But both were primarily administrators and neither had nor wished to have scientific training.

It is interesting to compare this quotation with one that follows in the next paragraph:

. . . the transformation of hospital nursing from a trade or hobby into a profession was not effected by rhetoric, but by business-like organization and ruthless discipline. She used all her advantages, intellect, social position, and "news value" and she succeeded. Her success places her among the greatest of pioneers in social medicine, not only of our country but of the whole world.

Strachey, although admitting Miss Nightingale's heroic deeds as a nurse, contended that all the activity to which she spurred Sidney Herbert between 1857 and 1860 so overworked him that he died soon afterwards. In essence, what both Greenwood and Strachey maintain is that it was proper for Miss Nightingale to be honored as a nurse, but that when she left that field, her behavior was held to be unacceptable.

Time and new approaches have revealed her very real contribution to the wider field of health planning and administration. And, in spite of these harsh judgments on her contributions to social reform, she was elected to fellowship in the Royal Statistical Society in 1858 and made an honorary member of the American Statistical Society in 1874.

Miss Nightingale began agitating for training in statistics at the universities because she was well aware of the double-edged rapier that statistics often represented. She maintained that members of Parliament used statistics mainly to "deal damnation" across the floor of the House. Her reason was that although the great majority of cabinet ministers, leaders of the army, government executives, and members of both Houses of Parliament had received a university education, "What has that university education taught them of the practical application of statistics?"

It must be remembered that in the three years following her return, the commission was formed and its report submitted; the statistical system of which I have spoken was designed and presented; *Notes on Hospitals* and *Notes on Nursing* were written; and, in 1860, the school of nursing at St. Thomas was founded.

While recognizing the danger of presenting a model of development created in another time and based on the post-Crimea activities of Miss Nightingale, one might nevertheless hypothesize that what was really happening was her moving through the three stages which deChardin claims to be the natural phases of complete personalization. The first stage is that of centration, which represents Miss Nightingale's early life when she was discovering herself, her profession, and her role. The second is decentration, post-Crimea, where the self becomes involved in ever and ever wider circles in a relationship to the outside world. Finally, there is supercentration, which requires the concern for the world to be wedded to the jump of faith.

DeChardin crystallizes these phases into: 1) unification of self within our two selves; 2) union of our own being with other beings who are our equals; and 3) subordination of our life to a cause greater than ours. "To tell the truth," deChardin says, "I see the complete solution to the problems of self-realization to the direction of a Christian humanism." That epitomizes the life and work of Florence Nightingale.

But where does all this leave us lesser mortals in the present age? Few of us can aspire to the third step. To rephrase our personal/professional growth analogy and return to the problems presented in the beginning of this article: What is the stage that the "new nurse" finds herself in today: centration or decentration?

It is no secret that the professionalists are dictating professional policy at this time. Professional degrees at the baccalaureate and master's levels are prerequisites for doctoral programs, and at least one state plans to limit RN licensure to nurses with at least a baccalaureate. Somewhat in reaction to this policy, physicians, having lost their handmaidens, have created new types of assistants, offering them advanced technical education long denied nurses as nurses. As long as these training programs are under the control of and accredited by the medical profession, they will repeat the frustrations of past education in nursing. How long these well-trained physicians' assistants will remain physicians' assistants before they begin their own process of professionalization is anyone's guess. But their role in a changing system must, of necessity, be fashioned alongside that of the new nurse.

In the meantime, the health care delivery system is undergoing radical changes which we can view as an era of control preceding the even more substantive alterations that will come with compulsory health insurance. Every aspect of health care will be quite different in the future. It is difficult to determine all the implications of change, but it is doubtful if many of the present relationships among providers and patients, particularly those controlled by the private fee structure, will survive.

These changes will have an enormous impact on nursing, whether the practitioners consider themselves "new" or "old." Professional Standards Review Organizations, mandated by Federal law to be composed of physicians, are spending substantial amounts of money to try to shorten patients' length of stay in acute hospitals, but not one extra dime has been voted to finance visiting nursing organizations to care for these early discharges. Health Systems Agencies will undoubtedly recommend ambulatory care and home programs for their geographic area; again, there is no money to carry out these recommendations. The nurse on the Connecticut Hospital Cost Commission was almost replaced by a non-nurse, in spite of the fact that nursing care accounts for about 30 percent of the hospital budget. Where are the nurses when decisions are made about the design of new health care systems?

It is possible, of course, that this conflict between the professionalists and the synergists may be overstated. The real problem may be that, although the conflict exists, nurses are so engaged in their own professionalization that they do not see the importance of becoming involved in changing the mode of delivering health services.

It is for this reason that I have examined these issues in the light of our heritage. For, despite a string of victories in the skirmishes surrounding the definition of the "new nurse," we may end up by losing the war. In fact, I believe we are destined to do so unless there is a Nightingale-like concern for the broader involvement of nurses in the redesign of the health care delivery system, with particular emphasis on the human considerations that have always characterized the nursing profession. Otherwise, nurses, old and new, will remain slaves as usual—underpaid and unrecognized—filling in the gaps and reacting to the problems that are bound to be created by solutions fashioned *without* nursing involvement.

Perhaps, instead, the new nurses will become involved in the struggle to reform the whole health system. Then it may be said of them, as Woodham-Smith said of their founder in a somewhat different arena, "Army welfare and army education, army recreation, sports and physical training, the health services, all came into being as a result of the Crimea. The agony had been frightful, but it had not been useless.

"It might, almost, be called a happy ending."

For Further Reading

The late William J. Bishop spent the last seven years of his life, from September, 1954 to his untimely death in July, 1961, deeply involved in a book to be entitled: *Bio-Bibliography of Florence Nightingale*. It was completed by his assistant, Sue Goldie, in 1962. The monumental project required that they steep themselves in the 200 or more books, pamphlets and articles attributed to Florence Nightingale as well as her 12,000 or so letters. Much of this mass of material had been published but just as much had not. As Mr. Bishop stated on several occasions, no doubt explaining his motivation: "the popular legend of Florence Nightingale is being perpetuated, while her own writings are neglected, and her most important achievements forgotten. There is little understanding of her real message for today."

Bishop and Goldie's *Bio-Bibliography* therefore "attempts for the first time, to provide a complete annotated list of Florence Nightingale's printed writings." As they reveal, in Miss Nightingale's incredibly busy life she wrote a plethora of books, pamphlets, magazine articles, memoranda, prefaces, introductions and much else. The range of her interests, for example, included the expected such as nursing, army hygiene and sanitation and hospital administration but also the newly developed field of statistics, considering herself a disciple of the trail-blazing Adolphe Quetelet, and the more far-reaching topics such as Indian army and land reforms, philosophy, religion, sociology and even "the proper feeding of birds" and raising of an owl.

Much of what she wrote on these subjects and so many others, meanwhile, was privately printed and not easily accessible or readily available. For its listing and annotating alone then the *Bio-Bibliography* has been a major breakthrough in Florence Nightingale historiography. As stated in the Introduction: "the object of the book is to show the immense scope of Florence Nightingale's work and at the same time to enable the interested reader to locate and consult any particular work for himself." Included in the work, for example, are entire

sections on the following topics: Nursing, The Army, Indian and
Colonial Welfare, Hospitals, Statistics, Sociology, Memoirs and Tri-
butes, Religion and Philosophy, Miscellaneous Works (including a
number of untraced works listed in Sir Edward Cook's two-volume
Life of Florence Nightingale) and Selected Writings about Florence
Nightingale and Her Times.

In the case of the last of these, as might be expected, the authors
note that much of the work written about her is "secondary and
derivative, and there would be little value in an exhaustive list." Yet,
they still manage to include writings from the following groups—
clearly a list unmatched anywhere:

1. Contemporary writings about F.N. throwing light on the development
   of the Nightingale legend.

2. Contemporary diaries and histories which fill in the background to her
   life and work, especially in the Crimea.

3. Important biographies based on original research; and their translations
   into other languages.

4. Articles written to illuminate a particular aspect of Miss Nightingale's
   work or thought, and containing previously unpublished fragments or
   letters.

5. Biographies of the friends and colleagues of Miss Nightingale.

It is therefore highly recommended that all interested in Florence
Nightingale begin with a thorough examination of this valuable source.
Moreover, since Bishop and Goldie admit that their compilation
"is based on Sir Edward Cook's very extensive 'List of Printed Writings
of Florence Nightingale' which appears at the end of Volume II" and
also quite obviously on Mrs. Woodham-Smith's "Sources" (divided
into MSS, Government Publications, Writings by Miss Nightingale
and Authorities) it would behoove the researcher to continue any
further study of Florence with an examination of these two works
as well. The only serious biography since that of Woodham-Smith
has been Elspeth Huxley's *Florence Nightingale* (N.Y.: 1975) which
not surprisingly acknowledged its debt to Woodham-Smith and Cook.
Unfortunately, this well-illustrated book was not thought to have
broken any new ground so, while obviously well-written, it was never-

theless described by at least one reviewer as no more than "an attractive cocoa table volume."

Many other biographies have appeared of course—some have been responsible for the semi-mythical portrait mentioned earlier. Many others however, have striven for objectivity above all else. Eliza Pollard's *Florence Nightingale: The Wounded Soldier's Friend*, for example, appeared in 1891 (London) well before Miss Nightingale's death (1910) or the commissioned two volume biography by Cook in 1913. Others that preceded Cook were Sarah A. Tooley's *The Life of Florence Nightingale* (London: 1908) and Laura E. Richard's *Florence Nightingale: The Angel of the Crimea* (N.Y.: 1909). The Cook work prevailed of course in the years immediately after Miss Nightingale's death until the iconoclastic Lytton Strachey's *Eminent Victorians* (London: 1918) included a controversial portrait of her as a woman possessed by a demon. The strong reaction against it that followed led to a rash of favorable works: Margaret Tabor's *Florence Nightingale* (London: 1925), Mary Raymond Shipman Andrew's *A Lost Commander: Florence Nightingale* (Garden City, N.Y.:1929), Ida B. O'Malley's *Florence Nightingale 1820-1856* (London: 1931), Irene Cooper Willis' *Florence Nightingale: A Biography* (London:1931), Margaret L. Goldsmith's *Florence Nightingale: The Woman and the Legend* (London: 1937), Winifred Wilson's *Florence Nightingale: Soldier's Heroine* (London: 1940), Ramona Barth's *Fiery Angel: The Story of Florence Nightingale* (Coral Gables, Florida: 1945), Rowena Keys' *Florence Nightingale: The Angel of the Crimea* (N.Y.: 1946), W. Millman's *Florence Nightingale: The Lady of the Lamp* (London: 1946).

In 1951, meanwhile, Mrs. Cecil Woodham-Smith was given the privilege of using many of the Verney-Nightingale papers to which Sir Edward Cook and many others did not have access. The result was her popular and well-reviewed *Florence Nightingale 1820-1910* (London and New York). Other frequently-quoted works of the 50's and 60's were those by Lucy Seymer who, in addition to her popular earlier *History of Nursing* (1933) also produced *Florence Nightingale* (London: 1950) and *Selected Writings of Florence Nightingale* (London: 1954) and Zachary Cope with a uniquely different approach as seen in *Florence Nightingale and the Doctors* (London: 1958) and *Six Disciples of Florence Nightingale* (London: 1961). But, the most unique and effective perspective pursued during these years can be found in Mildred E. Newton's unpublished Stanford University dissertation entitled *Florence Nightingale's Philosophy of Life and Education*.

Fortunately, however, the Newton treatise is used skillfully by Evelyn R. Barritt in the development of her arguments for one of the best articles of the 1970's: "Florence Nightingale's Values and Modern Nursing Education" (*Nursing Forum*, XII No. 1, 1973).

Not surprisingly, as we move into the late 60's and early 70's, the most interesting book was one edited by the same Ms. Barritt. Entitled *Florence Nightingale: Her Wit and Wisdom* (Mt. Vernon, N.Y.: 1975), it revealed a much-overlooked side—that of her own words and what wealth can be found within. Little has appeared in monograph form since the Woodham-Smith biography, however, there has been a steady outpouring of fine articles in recent years. Many of the best have been included in this volume. Unfortunately, one of the best, the Barritt article could not easily be accomodated to the format of this work. Other contributions by many of the selected authors, meanwhile, are also worth perusing: they include several by William Bishop, especially his "Florence Nightingale's Letters" (*AJN* 5, 1957 and *Nursing Mirror* 57, 1957); and Whittaker and Olesen's "Faces of Florence Nightingale" (*Human Organization* 23, Summer, 1964).

The best and/or most interesting of the articles that remain, meanwhile, are headed by two commemorative Florence Nightingale issues—the April, 1954 *International Nursing Review* and *RN* Magazine in May, 1970. The best articles from the former are Ellen Broe's "Florence Nightingale and her International Influence" and Evelyn C. Pearce's "The Influence of Florence Nightingale on the Spirit of Nursing." The latter issue featured not only the Isler article used in this book but also Bernice L. Shaw's "Florence Nightingale: Kaiserswerth Revisited." Among the others ranging back to her death, the articles worthy of note include: Stephen Paget's "Florence Nightingale" for the *Dictionary of National Biography* (1912); Leslie Shane's "Forgotten Passage in the Life of Florence Nightingale" (*Dublin Review*, 161, 1917); Rosalind Nash's defenses—"Florence Nightingale According to Mr. Strachey" (*The Nineteenth Century*, February, 1928) and "I Knew Florence Nightingale" (*Listener*, July 14, 1937); J. C. Mantripp's intriguing "Florence Nightingale and Religion" (*London Quarterly and Holborn Review*, July, 1932); Laura E. Richards' "Letters of Florence Nightingale" (*Yale Review: A National Quarterly*, 24, 1935); and numerous articles by Mrs. Woodham-Smith and Lucy Seymer in the 1950's. The late 1960's and 1970's brought forth several entries by behavioral scientists (such as Whittaker and Olesen and Donald Allen), on the one hand, and articles by medical people on the other: M.D. Lawrence Tinckler's "The Barracks at Scutari: Start of a Nursing

Legend" (*Nursing Times*, August 2, 1973), R.N. J. Elise Gordon's series
of articles on "The Work of Florence Nightingale" for a series about
Nurses and Nursing in Britain (*Midwife and Health Visitor*, August
through November, 1972), R.N. Jean Nelson's "Florence the Legend"
(*Nursing Mirror*, May 13, 1976) and two of the best by R.N. and Dean
of the University of San Diego School of Nursing, Irene Sabelberg
Palmer—"Florence Nightingale and the Salisbury Incident" (*Nursing
Research*, September-October, 1976) and "Florence Nightingale: Re-
former, Reactionary, Researcher" (*Nursing Research*, March-April,
1977). Additionally, the Barritt article, James Winchester's "Tough
Angel of the Battlefield" (*Today's Health*, May, 1967) and M. R. Grier's
"Contributions of the Passionate Statistician" (*Research in Nursing and
Health*, October, 1978) harken back interestingly enough, to the earlier
tradition.

The latter title, in fact, recalls the name coined by Sir Edward
Cook. In the same direction, soon after, Edwin W. Kopf wrote about
"Florence Nightingale the Statistician" for the American Statistical
Association (XV, 1918). Moreover, one decade later, the well-known
American pioneer of nursing in the Nightingale tradition, Mary Adelaide
Nutting, described Florence Nightingale as a Statistician" (*Public
Health Nurse*, 19, 1927) as well. As recently as 1978, Grier asks, as so
many have since Sir Edward Cook, "Is Florence Nightingale a Saint or
a Scientist?"

In conclusion, we note that even the most recent contributions
revert back to the same problems touched upon to one degree or
another by Sir Edward Cook and Mrs. Cecil Woodham-Smith. It is
clear therefore that the time has come for a new biographer to integrate the perspectives of the last three decades with the multiple
strengths of those two classic works for the production of 1980's version of Florence Nightingale's incredible life. Such a work, however,
should be firmly based on the foundation represented by the many
works that Mrs. Woodham-Smith listed as "Authorities" at the conclusion of her work: Baron Bunsen's *Memoirs* (London: 1868), *Constantinople During the Crimean War* by Lady Hornby (London, 1863),
The Autobiography of Elizabeth Davis, A Balaclava Nurse (London:
1857), *England and Her Soldiers* by Harriet Martineau (London:
1859), *Experiences of an English Sister of Mercy* by Margaret Goodman-
Smith (London: 1862), *Memoir of Sidney Herbert* by Lord Stanmore
(London: 1906), *The Life and Letters of Sir John Hall M.D.* by S. M.
Mitra (London: 1911), Evelyn Abbott and Lewis Campbell's two
volumes of *The Life and Letters of Benjamin Jowett* (London: 1897),

Memoirs of the Crimea by Sir Aloysius (London: 1897), *The Life, Letters and Friendships of Richard Monckton Milnes* by T. Wemyss Reid (London: 1890), Sir George Douglas' edited *Panmure Papers* (London: 1908), *Reminiscences* by Julia Ward Howe (Boston: 1900), *Sevastopol, Our Tent in the Crimea* and *Wanderings in Sevastopol* by Two Brothers (London: 1856), Alexis Soyer's *Soyer's Culinary Campaign* (London: 1857), *Life of Stratford de Redcliffe*, 2 volumes, by S. Lane Poole (London: 1888), M. C. M. Simpson's *Letters and Recollections of Julius and Mary Mohl* (London: 1887), F. Taylor's *Eastern Hospitals and English Nurses* (London: 1856), and of course, Reverend Osborne's *Scutari and its Hospitals* (London: 1855), William Howard Russell's *The British Expedition to the Crimea* (London: 1858) and Miss Nightingale's own abundant writings and family papers.

The above list is of course but a small sampling of many of the best works written about this incredible "woman for all seasons." But, whether one reads about her legend or about the work she accomplished in these or many others, the result should be the same—the realization best described by the man who started it all, William Howard Russell, the *London Times'* Crimean War Correspondent:

> Her faculty of conquering dominion over the minds of men was, above all, the force which lifted her from out of the ranks of those who are only "able" to the heights reached by those who are "great."